Intermittent Fasting for Women

The Ultimate Beginners Guide to Weight Loss, Burn Fat and Heal Your Body with Intermittent Fasting and Autophagy

Jenna Dawson

© Copyright 2019 Jenna Dawson

All rights reserved

Intermittent Fasting for Women

© Copyright 2019 Jenna Dawson All rights reserved.

Written by Jenna Dawson

First Edition

Copyrights Notice

No part of this book may be reproduced in any form or by any electronic or mechanical means, including information storage and retrieval systems, without written permission from the author.

Limited Liability

Please note that content of this book is based on personal experience and various information sources.

Although the author has made every effort to present accurate, up-to-date, reliable and complete information in this book, they make no representations or warranties with respect to the accuracy or completeness of the content of this book and specifically disclaim any implied warranties of merchantability or fitness for a particular purpose.

Your particular circumstances may not be suited to the example illustrated in this book; in fact, they likely will not be. You should use the information in this book at your own risk.

All trademarks, service marks, product names and the characteristics of any names mentioned in this book are considered the property of their respective owners and are used only for reference. No endorsement is implied when we use one of these terms.

This book is only for personal use. Please note the information contained within this document is for educational and entertainment purposes only and no warranties of any kind are declared or implied. Readers acknowledge that the author is not engaging in providing medical, dietary, nutritional or professional advice, or physical training.

Please consult a doctor, nutritionist or dietician, before attempting any techniques outlined in this book. Nothing in this book is intended to replace common sense or medical consultation or professional advice and is meant only to inform. By reading this book, the reader agrees that under no circumstances is the author responsible for any losses, direct or indirect, which are incurred as a result of the use of information contained within this document, including, but not limited to, errors, omissions, or inaccuracies.

Table of Contents

Introduction 10

Chapter 1 13

    What is Intermittent Fasting (IF)? 14

    History of intermittent fasting 15

    How does intermittent fasting work? 16

    Two IF states: Fed Vs. Fasted 16

    Fat-Adaptation 18

    How is IF different from dieting? 19

Chapter 2 23

    Why change your eating patterns? 24

    Does IF affect behavior? 25

    Health benefits of Intermittent Fasting 27

    Therapeutic benefits of Intermittent Fasting 31

    3 famous IF schedules 31

    Strategies of IF that proved most beneficial for women 38

    How to get started with intermittent fasting? 46

Chapter 3 49

    Design your own IF program 50

    Protocols necessary to succeed in intermittent fasting 52

    Significance of fluids during intermittent fasting 55

    Helpful tips for intermittent fasting 58

    How to use IF for muscle gain? 63

    Common mistakes to avoid during intermittent fasting 65

  Precautionary measures for intermittent fasting 71

  Female hormonal balance and intermittent fasting 74

  How does IF affect women differently than men? 75

Chapter 4 79

  When should women avoid intermittent fasting? 80

  Pros and cons of IF for women 81

  7-Day Intermittent Fasting guide for beginners 81

  Is exercise safe for women during IF? 91

Chapter 5 97

  Why is autophagy important for women? 98

  Keys to improve general health 101

  How does intermittent fasting prevent cancer? 107

  IF makes healthy eating simpler and easier 109

Chapter 6 111

  Tips to ease through intermittent fast 112

  Research-proven advantages of IF for women 114

  Reviews from women who practiced intermittent fasting 118

  Women who tried intermittent fasting for a week 118

  Woman who tried intermittent fasting for 8 months 119

Conclusion 123

  Final words on Intermittent Fasting for women 124

Introduction

World itself bears witness to the fact that many fitness and health trends have come and gone. Some catch the attention of the people and stay in trend for long periods of time like yoga while some of them draw immediate attention but lose the charm over time because of difficulty levels or side-effects. Everyone wants to be healthy, fit and wants to look attractive. And to do this, some people adopt the way of exercising and workouts while some people follow strict diet plans. In both scenarios, the purpose is to achieve goal weight, increase physical health and develop a peaceful state of mind.

Diets are pretty common in this day and age. They are more popular than any other weight-loss techniques. Men and women of all ages indulge in dieting but a majority of them ends up with nutritional deficiencies and with worse health condition than before. Diets limit the calorie intake of the day and this makes it difficult for you to meet the nutritional needs of the body. And this is where fasting comes in!

Fasting is actually the most popular and widely known technique known to humans for hundreds of centuries now. In some parts of the world, it is followed as a religious obligation like Christianity and Islam; while in others it is used as a natural and easy weight-loss tool. It can be used as both and humans all over the world can profit from this natural technique; no matter from which culture or race they belong to.

One of the most popular, easy and healthy fitness trends is *'intermittent fasting'*. By following this technique, you will not only lose weight and burn the fats but you will also nourish and heal your body. In other words, it is the healthiest way of losing weight known to man yet. It is also the easiest technique since it doesn't require extremely tough gym workouts or mind tormenting hunger levels. Anyone can apply this technique to their lives, because it doesn't need special efforts or time. *It is most beneficial for women* because they do not have any extra time while juggling work and home duties. Intermittent fasting is proven the most effective and most commonly adopted fitness technique by women all over the world.

Chapter 1

What is Intermittent Fasting (IF)?

The word 'Intermittent' has a literal meaning of 'occurrence at non-continuously and at irregular intervals'. Fasting means to 'abstain from a certain activity for a defined period of time'. 'Intermittent fasting' simply implies refraining from eating food for a certain defined time. There are two aspects regarding intermittent fasting:

- *Fasting window* – Period of time in which you abstain from eating.
- *Feeding window* – Period of time in which you are allowed to eat.

Fasting window is defined by you and you decide which hours of the day or which days of the week you can easily fast. If you are comfortable with a daily fast then you define major hours of the day as your 'fasting window'. During your fasting window, you are not allowed to eat anything. Anyway, there's no limit on fluid intake though. You can drink fluids as much you want during your fast. The best and suitable drinks for fasting will be discussed later.

Feeding window is known as those hours of the day when you are not under a fast and you can eat anything you want in this window. Unlike diets, there is no restriction on what to eat. As long as you eat healthy and fresh, you can have just about anything. During the feeding window, you meet the nutritional needs of your body and make up for the nutrition and energy that you took from it.

'Feeding window' has a range between 8 to 12 hours depending upon your stamina. Usually, it's a good practice to start with a long feeding window and shorter fasting window and then you gradually increase your fasting window and decrease the feeding window. Intermittent fasting (IF) is an eating pattern where your body cycles between periods of fasting and eating: so, this concept is based on voluntary abstinence from food for certain periods of time. Humans are designed and are well able to perform intermittent fasts. Intermittent fasting is a technique that anyone can implement as well as alter or change according to his/her routine. It focuses on stabilizing the times of eating which helps the body the body to get maximum energy out of a meal.

It is not the only weight-loss program out there but it is the healthiest one. Other weight-loss programs can include extreme starvation and deprivation from healthy fats, but Intermittent Fasting is the only weight-loss technique that focuses on providing nourishment and health to your body.

History of intermittent fasting

Humans have been fasting for thousands of years. Sometimes they did it due to religious obligations and sometimes just because there wasn't enough food. In the early histories of humankind, when there was a shortage of food, people used to perform extended fasts. They did not have access to an abundance of food and had food barely enough to survive. That is why; 'intermittent fasting' holds the title of the most ancient food practice in human history.

Now, although we live in a world where we see abundance of food, still a large population deliberately avoids eating food for longer periods and the intent is to lose weight. Researchers have conducted numerous studies and surveys and have found that tons of thousands of people from all around the world practice intermittent fasting on a weekly basis. Some religions put an obligation on its followers to fast while majority of people are in a race to lose fat mass, shedding extra pounds and thus improve their body composition.

It is true that IF is now gaining popularity in weight-loss and bodybuilding communities, but it is not a new technique. It has been used my humans since the 1900s and it therapeutically treated many diseases like epilepsy, diabetes and also obesity. In modern day of time, intermittent fasting is attracting the attention of scientists as well as celebrities alike. While the scientists are conducting extensive researches on it benefits and using it as a medical aid in the health field, celebrities are looking for effective and best ways to attain a perfect and inspiring shape of body.

How does intermittent fasting work?

Our body can handle extended periods of not eating. Human bodies have the natural ability to transition between the hunger state and the full state. When we don't eat for a long period of time, the processes going inside our body change. When we eat our body starts to work on digesting it and storing the energy received through the meal. When we are hungry, our body starts to take energy from those stored fats.

When we are fasted for a specific period of time, our blood sugar and insulin levels face a reduction in their levels. It is normal because it pushes our body to thrive from existing resources present inside our bodies. Researches have shown that fasting helps to protect against diseases like heart diseases, diabetes, cancer and Alzheimer's disease. Therefore, when in a fasted state, you shouldn't worry that you shouldn't worry that it will affect your health.

In order to understand how intermittent fasting works, two states have to be understood first. The two states are – the fed state and the fasted state. By understanding these states, we get to know that how our bodies keep functioning well regardless of the fact that our stomachs are empty or full.

Two IF states: Fed Vs. Fasted

In the *Fed state*, the body is undergoing process of digesting and absorbing food. The state begins when you start eating and can last from three to five hours after that. In fed state, your body shows elevated levels of insulin, and this acts as a signal for your body to store the excess amounts of calories. This storage takes place in the fat cells. During the time with high insulin levels, the process of fat burning comes to a stop and the body shifts towards burning glucose from your last meal instead.

Then a state called *post-absorptive* state comes, which lasts about 8 to 12 hours after the last meal. After that the body enters the **Fasted state**. In the *Fasted state*; body is not processing any meal and the levels of insulin are low. This induces a mobilization of stored body fat presiding inside the body in the fat cells, and starts to burn these fats for providing energy to the body. In this state, the body can burn the fat that was first inaccessible to it during the fed state.

Staying hungry for a specific duration of time helps you with hundreds of things. When you eat a meal, your body is under 'fed state' and is just processing the meal you just ate. After a few hours pass and the food is completely digested, it goes into a mid-stage where you don't feel hungry but you haven't eaten anything else yet. You can call this an intermediate state. After 8 to 12 hours from your last meal, a state comes called 'fasted state' when you feel hungry and you are under a fast. In this state, your body needs to re-gain the fuel to work but it doesn't find any energy being provided to it. So, it starts to look for energy sources inside the body. It starts to go towards the fat cells where fats from your previous meals have been stored. The body is designed to store some amount of fat from every meal in order to regain energy at the time when it is needed. Thus, because of low insulin levels now the body has entered into a fat-burning state and it starts to burn the fats present inside the body. This is beneficial in hundreds of ways. It will not only get rid of the excess fat from you, but will also get rid of any toxins present inside a body.

The toxins can be anything harmful present in your body. It can be dysfunctional cell or a cell that is damaged and is not performing well. Removal of such cells is very necessary when we talk about maintaining health. So, you have to be under the 'fasted state' so that your body can initialize the burn-off state. Intermittent fasting provides you a convenient way to enter into the fasted state and get rid of all excess fats, calories and damaged cells. Many health-practitioners and doctors advise their patients to start fasting for this purpose. They believe that health will improve if they fast because of this quality of intermittent fasting.

Fat-Adaptation

Nature has given humans the ability to fuel their bodies with stored body-fat instead of glucose and extra calories. Just a little **time and practice** is needed to achieve the goal of regulating your metabolism based on existing resources in your body and let your body to adapt fat-burning pathways. This practice is called *Fat-adaptation*. It includes improving your body's sensitivity to lower insulin levels and promoting mobilization of the fat from fat cells, so that the body leans towards extracting energy from fat reserves inside the body instead of depending on constant fat resources being given to it externally through food.

At first a person might perceive that this fasting technique is hard since it requires you to stay away from food in some portions of the day. But it is actually a totally wrong perception. ***IF does not stop or change what you eat; it just changes when you eat it.*** It has already been proven that eating too much or having large meals slows your metabolism, increases laziness and reduces productivity of a person. Eating small portions of food at appropriate times of the day not only gives you higher energy levels but also boosts your metabolism and thus your body keeps getting healthier.

Thus, in order to burn the existing fat in your body, fasted state has to be achieved. Your body will itself take energy from calories and fats already presiding in your body and that's how the fat is naturally burned away from our bodies. Fasting puts the body in a state of burning fat and we cannot enter the fasted state until 8 to 12 hours from the last meal. This time is different for everyone since it depends on the metabolism rate. It is important to practice the learning curve and you will get your body on track naturally.

How is IF different from dieting?

Intermittent fasting is *not a diet* in the conventional sense; in fact, it is a pattern of eating. It is a technique where you schedule your meals so that you and your body can get the most out of them.

Unlike diet plans, Intermittent Fasting does not focus on what to eat and what not to eat. This phenomenon puts emphasis on when to eat so that it may prove beneficial to your body. Despite what some people may think, intermittent fasting is a fairly easy technique. Studies have been conducted in this regard and majority of people have reported that they have higher energy levels during the fasting periods of the day.

The biggest difference between dieting and fasting is that dieting makes you stick to specific foods only and intermittent fasting keeps the options open for your stomach. You can enjoy whole meals filled with nutrition, protein and even some healthy fats.

Diets like low-carb diets make you eat empty carbs and this does not provide any nutrition to your body. Human's bodies specifically female body needs all possible nutrition to stay healthy and fit. And if you restrict your food intake to only a few foods, you will never be able to achieve a healthy and sound body.

Another difference between the two is *Effectiveness* in same time period. Dieting has proved very beneficial for some individuals and they claim they lost about 10 or 15lbs in one week. But this comes at a heavy cost - losing sleep, facing anger problems due to starvation and an overall bitterness to the personality and nature.

This happens because you are not naturally allowing the body to reduce fat; in fact, you are forcing your body to go through states which it generally won't go through.

On the other hand, Intermittent Fasting takes a much natural and consistent approach towards weight loss. It might take more time than conventional dieting, but it won't take a negative toll on your mind or health. It won't induce anger or anxiety due to extreme hunger levels; instead it will take a rather slower approach to get rid of the access fat from your body naturally.

One major difference between the two is of **Consistency**. You can never follow diet plans more than a few months or even a year.

After that, you get annoyed and go right back to your old eating habits and gain the lost weight back in no time. This is something that pushes people in severe depression and they end up gaining more weight than they originally had. IF offers an easy to follow and convenient method to achieve your goal weight. You can make a permanent lifestyle out of it, adapt it as long as you want and you never have to give it up because of difficulty. It is a very simple technique, does not require much effort or time.

Flexibility is another difference between the two. Dieting specifically tells you what foods to eat and avoid what foods.

Everyone has to follow the same instructions, eat specific foods, tediously counting and limiting calorie intake. It is not at all flexible, meaning you cannot enjoy a pizza or a piece of cake every once in a while, because you will gain back the lost pounds. IF on the other hand is flexible and every individual can tailor and customize it according to his own self. You can set eating times according to your will and ease, you don't have to face extreme restrictions on what foods to eat. You are allowed to eat just about everything; you just have to follow a healthy schedule of when to eat.

Chapter 2

Why change your eating patterns?

The reason why intermittent fasting is so widely popular is that it doesn't require abstaining from food; it just demands healthier eating time patterns. Isn't it better to just eat at specific times instead of putting yourself through the miseries of extreme dieting rules? Instead of worrying about fats in different foods and counting calories before eating and being unable to relish your favorite foods, just adjust the patterns of eating and still enjoy a healthy body weight. Just tweak your schedules of eating and the job is done. That simple!

Intermittent fasting is the **simplest strategy** to lose weight. It doesn't put a stress toll on your mind and stomach because of staying hungry. It also doesn't demand drastic change in lifestyle or behavior. It is simple enough for anyone to actually implement it; yet so meaningful that it will really can make a difference. This phenomenon simply takes of excess weight from your body while keeping on the good weight on which helps you feel energetic throughout your day.

Diets are easy to contemplate but difficult to execute. The fast results of a diet appeal everyone, but when you really get into it, it becomes very tough very early. Suppose, you decide that you are going on a low-carb diet, a major portion of delicious and appealing foods have to be avoided. Also, after staying hungry for long durations, you have to force yourself to eat foods that you don't want to eat all the time. Whereas, in Intermittent Fasting, you are not restricted on choices of food, you are just challenged to maintain proper eating times and patterns. Thus, to conclude, diet requires the work than fasting. In a diet, you not only stay hungry, but also you don't get to eat what you like. But in Intermittent Fasting, you just have to follow a schedule of eating and never have to worry about what to eat and what not to eat. Therefore, ease of intermittent fasting is intriguing to lose weight. Because it is easy to contemplate as well as execute. It also provides a huge range of health benefits that a diet can never provide. Unlike a diet, IF doesn't snatch away nutrition from your body, that's why it keeps you healthy. Moreover, a diet requires a massive change in lifestyle and eating habits. Intermittent Fasting is easy to implement and never demands huge alterations and modifications in lifestyle.

Does IF affect behavior?

Behaviors classify into two categories- health behaviors and personality behaviors. Let's see how does Intermittent Fasting affect both behaviors and does it enhance the quality of life or not?

Health behaviors: Intermittent fasting has proved to help improve and modify different health behaviors like calorie intake, energy-expenditure and sleep. Calorie intake means how much you eat and energy expenditure refers to how much you move.

A balance between both of them is necessary to provoke a healthy lifestyle and an active body. If you eat too much and move less, it will only affect your health negatively and might act as the biggest drawback to your extra weight. The reverse of this case is also true.

If you exert a lot of energy during the day but then have an extremely heavy and large meal, this will also slow your metabolism rate and as a result you will gain weight. The last meal before sleeping must be a small meal so that your body can digest it before you sleep and this will allow your body to enter a state of fasting.

This nightly fasting will decrease your calorie intake and will produce a significant decrease in weight. In return, this improves: Energy levels and sleep satisfaction.

Intermittent fasting also reduces untimely snacks during the night and decreases the nighttime intake of food which enhances the quality of sleep. Poor sleep quality leads towards risk of obesity, diabetes and many heart-related diseases. Therefore, Intermittent Fasting plays a significant role in improving the health behaviors thus giving you a healthier lifestyle.

Personality Behaviors: When you suddenly put your body through huge gaps of food intake during dieting and do not provide necessary nutrients like protein and healthy carbs, your body enters a state of constant exhaustion and fatigue. This induces a state of stress on your body and indirectly it's you who faces the stress and exhaustion.

The will to work is reduced, your energy levels drop and you find yourself in the mood to lie down and do minimize your activities. Not moving enough and lying around makes your body habitual of the constant rest state and makes you lazy. You don't want to walk, talk, work or participate in social activities. You start becoming an introvert and that's how your whole personality shifts due to the drastic change in your diet.

Intermittent Fasting presents the best solution for this. Intermittent Fasting does not induce massive and drastic changes in your diet plans. It slowly and steadily brings your body towards a schedule to eat at healthy times. This allows your body to extract maximum energy out of it and you feel energized for longer durations of time. You stay healthy, happy and active. You start to work more, stay more active thus your physical as well as mental health improves.

This fasting technique which defines windows of eating, not only improves your mental health which accounts for personality behaviors. It also puts your body on a healthier path, and with passage of time you learn the best eating patterns that suit your lifestyle and personality. Intermittent Fasting works for every person because it allows the ease of implementation. If your job requires you to work all night and you sleep in the day, Intermittent Fasting offers a relaxed schedule to maintain suiting your requirements. You can define your own window of eating and adjust accordingly.

Health benefits of Intermittent Fasting

Numerous studies conducted link Intermittent Fasting to substantial benefits for one's body, as well as the brain. The following list includes some of the most important evidence-backed advantages of Intermittent Fasting:

- *Weight loss and burning belly fat*: A major cause behind people, and especially women, taking up Intermittent Fasting is their concern for and the desire to lose weight and burn as much belly fat as possible. Since, Intermittent Fasting requires one to eat fewer meals, it automatically reduces the calorie intake. Furthermore, it enhances the body's metabolic rate by 3.6 – 14% by lowering insulin levels and stimulating growth hormones, which ultimately work towards breaking down carbohydrates and body fat and speeding its use for energy. Thus, Intermittent Fasting effectively tackles both sides of the calorie equation – decreasing the intake with fewer meals and increasing the burnout with an increased metabolic rate.

    A 2014 scientific literature review showed 3 – 8% weight loss over 0.75 to 6 months due to intermittent fasting. A loss of 4 – 7% of waist circumference was also reported, which indicates loss of belly fat. In fact, one such study proved that Intermittent Fasting was better compared to continuous calories restriction as it resulted in lesser muscle lost.

- *Reduced insulin resistance and Lower risk of diabetes:* There is no doubt diabetes is a serious health condition and one that has become increasing common over the past few decades, particularly type-2 diabetes. Type-2 diabetes occurs essentially when the body's blood sugar level rises above normal and the body has a higher insulin resistance, which means the insulin is not being used properly. Consequently, anything that would help lower this insulin resistance should eventually contribute to lowering one's blood glucose level and prevent (or protect against) type 2 diabetes. Intermittent Fasting, in this regard, has actually been proven to result in notable blood sugar level reduction.

Studies have shown that Intermittent Fasting lead to a 20 – 31% decrease in insulin resistance, while decreasing the blood glucose by 3 – 6%. Additionally, according to a study conducted on diabetic rats, Intermittent Fasting appears to protect against and prevent damage to the kidney which happens to be one of the biggest complications of diabetes. Based on a 2014 review paper in the ***Translational Research*** journal, overweight and obese adults who observed intermittent fasting showed a reduction in diabetes markers i.e. insulin sensitivity. All this implies that people at risk of becoming a victim to type-2 diabetes can use Intermittent Fasting to protect against it.

- *Improved heart health:*
  Heart disease happens to be one of the leading causes of death in the world. Such diseases are more or less caused by the unhealthy eating habits of our generation. Numerous risk factors are linked to increased or decreased risk of heart disease. A 2016 review claims that intermittent fasting in both humans and livestock could result in reduced blood pressure, cholesterol, heart rate and triglycerides. By the end of the day, anything unhealthy directly affects the heart and it is important to keep your heart in a healthy condition.
- *Improved brain health:* Brain health is not something that should be taken lightly and efforts must be made to ensure

that an individual is physically, and more importantly, mentally sound. And intermittent fasting goes a long way in this regard. Metabolic features are known to be extremely important for brain health and, as previously mentioned, intermittent fasting has proven to improve several of these features, including reduction in oxidative stress, inflammation, insulin resistance and blood sugar levels – all of which are associated with neurological conditions. Several studies conducted on mice have shown the positive results of intermittent fasting as it has boosted the growth of their nerve cells which has improved their brain function. One study which compared the learning ability and memory of mice on an intermittent fasting diet and mice with free access to food showed that the former was better at retaining as well as acquiring new information. Intermittent fasting has also been known to increase brain-derived neurotrophic factor (BDNF) levels, a brain hormone the deficiency of which could lead to depression and several other neurological disorders. In fact, certain animal studies have discovered that the risk of neurological disorders, such as Alzheimer's disease, Parkinson's disease, Huntington's disease and strokes can be reduced with the help of intermittent fasting.

- ***Prevention of Alzheimer's disease:*** as stated above, intermittent fasting is beneficial for mental health but its impact on the world's most common neurogenerative disease like Alzheimer's is even more crucial. Alzheimer's disease is an incurable condition, which means preventing it from occurring in the first place is critical.

Intermittent fasting studies conducted on rats showed a delay in the early onset Alzheimer's and even decreased its severity. In addition to that, a series of case reports brought to light the fact that a lifestyle intervention that included

intermittent fasting resulted in considerable improvement in the disease's symptoms in 9 out of 10 patients.
- *Anti-aging benefits and protection against chronic diseases:* one of the factors contributing to aging and chronic diseases is oxidative stress. This, basically, refers to an imbalance between the antioxidants in one's body and the free radicals. Research carried out has shown Intermittent Fasting to boost the body's resistance to oxidative stress, thus, providing anti-aging benefits. Moreover, Intermittent Fasting helps guard against inflammation – a major cause behind several common diseases.
- *Reduced risk of cancer:* cancer, a terrible disease resulting from uncontrollable growth (mutation) of cells, can be prevented with intermittent fasting. Intermittent Fasting's effective impact on a body's metabolic rate (as discussed earlier) has been known to reduce the risk of having cancer. Animal studies have come up with promising evidence of prevention of cancer through intermittent fasting as they have shown that such restrictive diets delayed the onset of tumors in animals who observed it. A study on human cancer patients who observed intermittent fasting showed a reduction in various chemotherapy side effects.

Given the fact that obesity is a major health marker for several tumors, the weight loss aspect of Intermittent Fasting could also be a contributor to the reduced risk of cancer. Finally, intermittent fasting can also help prevent cancer through its effect on insulin levels and inflammation, which are among the various biological factors associated with cancer.

- *Extension of Lifespan:* one of the most intriguing applications of intermittent fasting yet is its potential to extend the lifespan and help one live longer.
  Animal researches, particularly the studies on rats, show that intermittent fasting contributes to lifespan extension

in the same way as a continuous calorie restriction does. One study showed a dramatic increase of lifespan by 83% in the rats which fasted compared to those who did not.

Therapeutic benefits of Intermittent Fasting

Physical benefits – Intermittent fasting is being authenticated as an aid for preventing seizures and brain damage caused by seizures. It also gives a healing hand in curing arthritis (inflammation in joints). It also helps to reduce the toxic effects of chemotherapy and alternate day fasting also reduces the chances of cancer.

Spiritual benefits – Fasting is known to be a spiritual practice in many religions and culture all across the globe. All religions are different and unique, yet all of them share and promote fasting as a healing and healthy practice. A healthy body makes the soul healthy and peaceful; this is perhaps the most important beneficial spiritual aspect. Thus, if you are looking for regaining the spirituality of your soul and bringing peace to your inner-self; intermittent fasting is the best of all options.

Psychological benefits – When you are fasting, you are constantly controlling your mind and are consciously choosing not to eat. This trains your brain muscles and helps them to strengthen.

After learning how to control your mind, you slowly develop a power to control further aspects of your life too. Recent studies have shown that Intermittent Fasting helped women to increase sense of achievement, control, pride and self-esteem. And when you finally break your fast and enter into the feeding window; you gain an incredible sense of life, gratitude for food and nutrition and feel blissful because of nourishment of body.

3 famous IF schedules

There are many ways of integrating intermittent fasting. Three most common ones include:

Daily Intermittent fasting – *A fasting schedule that has a daily window of feeding and fasting windows. You define these windows as you want. Begin from short windows and slowly progress to large time windows.*

Weekly Intermittent fasting – *A fasting schedule that requires you to specify 2 or 3 days of the week to fast. Start off by fasting two days of the week, strengthen and make your body habitual and then move towards 3 day fast in a week schedule.*

Alternative Day Intermittent fasting – *A fasting schedule which alternates between 24 hours of fasting and 24 hours of eating. This is not for beginners. People just getting introduced to Intermittent Fasting should not try this fasting. It is for only those who have mastered the above two fasting schedules and are looking for a tougher challenge.* These schedules are designed for individuals who want to go easy, simple and non-complex. Many of the readers and researchers look up for to-the-point understanding and implementation of these schedules. Therefore, a precise detail is described below for each one of these schedules.

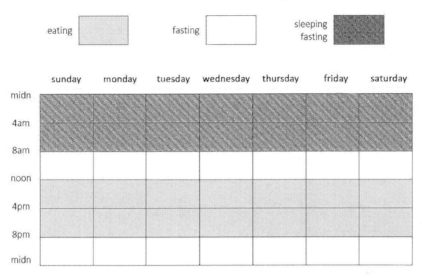

Daily intermittent fasting. The daily intermittent fasting schedule involves a 16-hour fasting period, which is then followed by an 8-hour feeding period. The 8-hour feeding window could be whatever suits one depending on their lifestyles – whether it starts 7am in the morning to 3pm in the afternoon or from 1pm to 9pm.

The first and foremost consideration is the feeding window's duration. If you are just a beginner and are just stepping into fasting lifestyle, then it's better for you to start from shorter fasting windows and longer feeding windows. For example, instead of a 16-hour fasting window, start with 12 or 13 hour fasting window.

This will help your body to adjust to the new changes and you will not over-exhaust yourself in the very beginning. When you see that you have built-up enough stamina and can easily undergo a 12-hour fasting window, slowly increase the fasting window and move it up by one hour. Now, you will practice this level of fasting and in this way slowly progress towards 16/8 fasting schedule.

As the name suggest, this routine is carried out every day, which makes it easier to get into the habit of a certain eating schedule.

All one needs is to learn when not to eat and the whole schedule is easily set in place. Despite the numerous pros, a possible disadvantage of the daily intermittent fasting model of intermittent fasting is that since there is a 16-hour fasting window, a meal or two is easily cut out every single day.

This means the body's weekly calorie intake goes down and the observer ends up losing weight. This, depending on one's goals, could be a pro or a con – pro for someone aiming at weight loss and a con for the one trying to maintain their calorie intake.

Maintaining a chart, like the one above, could help one in sticking to an assigned schedule.

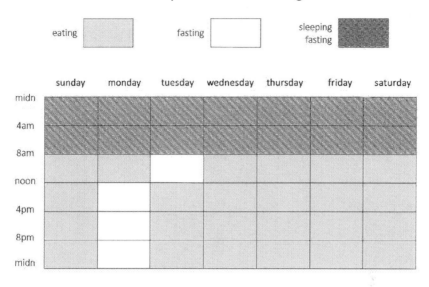

Weekly intermittent fasting. A preferred way to get on with intermittent fasting is to observe it just once every week. The weekly intermittent fasting has been linked to several of the benefits shared earlier in the book. Thus, even if the goal behind using this technique is not related to weight loss or cutting down calories, this method would still yield a positive outcome.

An example of weekly intermittent fasting would be to have lunch, say at 12pm, on Sunday and then fast until the lunch time on Monday. This would give a 24-hour fasting period each week. This technique would allow one to reap the benefits of fasting while still eating every day of the week. Given the fact that only 2 meals within a weak are skipped, it is unlikely that one would lose weight.

Hence, if the objective is to lose weight, weekly intermittent would not be the best option. But if the losing the calories is not an issue and the aim is to simply maintain a healthy lifestyle, then this technique is the way to go. One of the biggest pros of the weekly intermittent fasting is that it helps shatter the "mental barrier of fasting". This means that if one has never experienced fasting before, observing fasting using this technique would help one ease into it without emotionally disturbing them. A sample chart, like the one above, could be used to plan out weekly Intermittent Fasting.

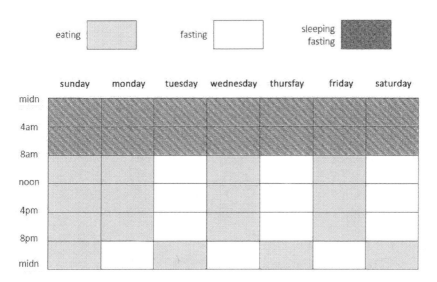

Alternate Day intermittent fasting. Alternate day intermittent fasting, as the name suggests, refers to longer fasting windows on alternate days in a week. In alternate day Intermittent Fasting, for instance, if one eats dinner on Sunday, he or she would then fast for 24 hours and have their next meal on Monday evening. Tuesday would be a feeding period and one would eat all day and then start the next 24-hour fasting cycle after having dinner on Tuesday evening, and so on. This method allows one to have at least one meal per day and still enjoy the benefits of long fasting periods on a consistent basis. As you can see; this fasting schedule is harder and longer than all others. In this fasting schedule you have to stay on a fast for 24 hours and then for the next 24 hours you can eat.

This is not best suitable for beginners. This can prove extremely hard for you if you are just stepping into the fasting world. Always make sure to start-off easy and slowly progress your way to the top. The chart above is an example of Alternate Day Intermittent Fasting.

An advantage of alternate day intermittent fasting is that it increases the benefits of fasting, hypothetically, compared to daily intermittent fasting because it involves having longer fasted state time as compared to the latter. Practically, however, it is not as suitable. This method makes it extremely difficult to have enough feast days to make up for the fasted days.

This way of intermittent fasting is, therefore, not too common in the real world and is mostly used by bodybuilders and professionals who can take easily take up this type of fasting.

General public especially women with already sensitive insulin levels, usually find it very hard to manage this fasting schedule.

Especially of you have irregular eating patterns, do not try this schedule at first. Start with something that is doable for you and once you get comfortable with that, you can increase the fasting or feeding window and move on.

Note:

The best option is to try and incorporate daily and weekly intermittent fasting styles. Start-off with weekly fasting schedule which requires you to fast two days a week. Once you are comfortable with weekly schedule, progress your way to daily fasting. Practice observing it once a week or once a month and then decide for yourself, which of these IF schedules suit you the best.

Strategies of IF that proved most beneficial for women

There are many techniques and methods out there for intermittent fasting. But it is important to note that not every one of them is suitable for women. Some require extreme and drastic measures like staying hungry for extraordinarily long periods of time. This can disturb the diet plan for women and also might disturb the hormonal balance and may start hundreds of other problems.

There are some types of Intermittent Fasting which are specifically designed for bodybuilders and men. Following those types can severely impact the health of women because they are too tough to implement. That is why; the types of intermittent fasting that have been proven beneficial for women are listed below:

1) The 5:2 intermittent fasting:

The 5:2 fasting method is most popular and the most common intermittent fasting method. It is called the '5:2' because you eat 5 days of the week in a normal and regular pattern. While the remaining two days of the week, you limit your calorie intake. The limit is in between 500 to 600 calories per day.

Again, it is not a diet, so you are not restricted on what to eat and what to avoid. You can choose anything that you want to eat, you just have to limit it's intake to a fixed number of calories. Meaning eating small portions at one time and increase the number of meals if you want to. It all depends on you; you are the one in the driving seat and can make decisions according to your routine and work schedule.

How to implement this method? First of all, think about your schedule and busiest days of the week. You can opt not to fast on those days so that it doesn't pressure you or your diet. So, choose the 5 days you don't want to fast on and eat regularly as you used to on those days. Then, pick two days on which you can fast easily and they should have an average gap between them.

For example, if you are choosing Tuesday as day one of your fast, then pick Friday as the second day. This will allow an even gap between your fast that is a gap of three days between each fasting day. Whatever days you choose, there must be at least one or two day gap between them.

After choosing your fasting days, suiting your lifestyle and routine, the second step is to think of dividing your calorie intake for your days of fasting. Meaning that since you have 500 calorie intake allowed, divide them into two meals of 250 calories or you can increase the number of meals by further shrinking the size of the meal. This will keep you active and energized throughout the day besides the fact that you are fasting. Do not take one meal of 500 calories because after 8 to 12 hours you will feel hunger levels striking very high and you will be unable to eat anything since you have already consumed your calorie intake of the day. This will leave you lethargic and lazy for the rest of the day.

So, either you can have three small meals consisting of breakfast, lunch and dinner. Or have two slightly bigger meals; lunch and dinner only. It is normal to feel hungry and weaker on first few fasts, but your body will very soon adjust to new changes and you will get used to fast days and won't affect you that much.

In conclusion, this is a type of intermittent fast that you can customize according to your own self. Every woman can fix the days suiting her and her schedule and thus every woman out there can benefit from this method of fasting.

How is it beneficial for women? 5:2 is extremely easy and simple to implement. Every woman can tailor this fasting method according to her own self. Women with kids and work can choose differently and housewives can choose differently. It provides you the flexibility that no other diet will ever provide you. It spares you from tedious calculations of daily calorie intake. It does not prohibit you from eating your favorite foods.

The only condition is to not go overboard with them and amalgamate healthy and nutritious foods in your diet too. So that, your body keeps receiving the necessary nutrition supply and you can lose weight without losing patience or health.

Advantages:

- You don't have to follow calorie restriction every day, thus making it easier to implement.
- Many studies have shown that regular calorie restriction helps to lose weight more efficiently.
- Women with higher insulin levels can benefit from it because this fasting method lowers the insulin levels in the body.
- It also improves the sensitivity to insulin.
- It reduces fat mass without affecting muscle mass.
- It also helps to reduce weight as well as inflammation in bodies.

2) Intermittent fasting with 8-hour eating window:

If you follow 8 hour eating window fasting, it means that your fasting window is of 16 hours and your feeding window is of 8 hours. It is also one of the simplest and easiest fasting methods and beneficial for women since it doesn't require full days of fasting. It just needs specifying which portion of the day to fast and in which portion eat. This is also an adaptable and adjustable fasting way and anyone can fix the hours according to their lifestyle and schedule. The most common practice followed by the practitioners of this technique is fast from dinner to lunch.

This only makes you skip breakfast and you also complete the fasting window without stressing your body too much. The key point of this fasting method is **Consistency**. If you do not follow the same schedule every day, staying hungry for 16 hours won't matter. Reason being you are not training your body to burn incessantly present fats inside the body. The body won't be able to learn your eating habits and thus it won't be able to make a decision when to burn the fats and when not to. It is because you are eating at inconsistent hours and are constantly changing your fasting and feeding windows.

Some women like to keep light exercising in their daily schedule. Strict diet plans followed with exercise is too much exhaustion for women's bodies. Therefore, this intermittent fasting technique helps women to maintain a fasting schedule, maintain a healthy and nutritious feeding schedule and also incorporate light exercising. Many women have reported that this technique has worked the best for them and they never stopped following it because of its excellent results in weight loss while maintaining a healthy body.

Those who are looking for how to start intermittent fasting are suggested to start from implementing this fasting method. It is the simplest and requires the least effort on the practitioner's end. It is not an extreme food deprivation technique, thus making it easy for the beginners to enter a healthy lifestyle.

How to implement this method? Simply select the 16-hour fasting window and 8 hour feeding window. This selection is based solely on your lifestyle and work schedule. If you have tough and tedious working hours during the day then choose the evening and night as your fasting window. And if you are a beginner and are looking for easiest way to start intermittent fasting, choose windows that make you skip breakfast. That way you can enjoy lunch and dinner and fast through the night. Again, this method is customizable according to anyone.

How is it beneficial for women? Women with extremely hard days and having busiest schedules are suggested to start from 14 hour fasting window and 10 hour feeding window. This might seem more doable and more practical to women since they have lower energy levels than men. Once you are comfortable with 14:10 hour window, move towards 16:8 hour window. *This is a huge convenience for women since they can start out slow and move further along according to their pace and stamina.*

Many other fasting ways like 24-hour fasting is not suitable for women. This technique is inspired by bodybuilders and weight-lifters. Since it requires extreme depravation of food for 24 hours and then heavy and full of protein meals for the next 24 hours helps body builders to achieve higher body mass and muscles.

Women cannot benefit from this technique at all. It may disturb their eating and sleeping schedules. That's why; 8 hour feeding intermittent fasting is extremely beneficial for women.

Advantages:

- Start according to your own pace and stamina.
- Best way of intermittent fasting for beginners.
- Customizable for every individual.
- Easy and simple to implement.
- No need for keeping track of calorie intake all the time.
- Saves busy women a lot of time and effort.
- Once beginner level is achieved, you can move to even longer fasting windows.
- Gives time to your body to adapt to the fasting schedule.
- Doesn't leave you feeling weak or low in energy.

3) Spontaneously skip the meals:

This is a non-scheduled type of fasting unlike above mentioned ways of fasting. While other ways of intermittent fasting require a schedule keeping and keeping track of fasting and feeding windows, this type of fasting is conducted whenever convenient.

For example, women who are free on weekends and don't have much activity on these days can skip the meals when they are not feeling hungry. Because your activity is lessened on the weekend, it is quite appropriate to lessen your food intake too.

This will automatically reduce the calorie count inside your body and you will lose weight without even trying. Skipping a meal or two spontaneously is also an intermittent fast.

Though spontaneous and unplanned, yet it benefits you the same way as a planned fast would. Suppose you are travelling and haven't found a healthy food spot, start a fast. And then when you reach your destination, you would already have burned a lot of fat and then by eating healthy foods, you will supply the nutrition to your body without giving it access calories.

Spontaneous fasting has proven very beneficial in many researches and studies. The human body is well-equipped to handle long periods of hunger and fasting, because this starts up the process of disintegration of stored body fats. When you skip a meal, your body doesn't get it resource of energy from outside. That's what forces it to decompose existing fat residing inside the fat cells. This is a very healthy approach towards weight loss and anyone can do it anytime, anywhere.

How is it beneficial for women? Have you been working all day and couldn't find time to prepare a meal and to eat it? You just performed a spontaneous intermittent fast! How does this help you? Your body has been taking its necessary fuel from fat reservoirs inside your body and unconsciously you have lost a bunch of calories. Your body practiced how to depend on its ownself in case when you skip a meal and next time when you skip a meal; it knows how to refuel the energy tank. Thus, unknowingly and without trying you removed some of the access from your body.

Advantages:
- Triggers the present at inside body.
- Burns the excess fat presiding in fat cells.
- Provides energy to your body while shedding off extra fat.

- No need of following schedules of eating and fasting.
- Unplanned and easy weight loss.

4) Reducing portions of food during the 'feeding-window':

This is an intermittent fasting technique which is implemented very slowly and steadily. This technique also doesn't require following any schedules. It just demands slowly reducing food portions when you are eating during your feeding-window.

This is an automatic technique of fasting; meaning by slowly reducing the daily calorie intake, you automatically come under intermittent fasting technique. It resembles the '5:2 intermittent fasting' because you limit your calorie intake during the fasting days. The difference is; you don't have to define the fasting days. Just simply reduce calorie intake and you won't really need to maintain schedules of fasting and non-fasting.

How to implement this method? The goal is to take your diet towards smaller meal portions. But the key-point is to not be rash and extra fast while doing so. This might leave the body dealing and coping with deficiencies. Therefore, be slow and gentle while doing so. Start by lessening the portion a tiny bit and work your way up to eating small portions of food and still satisfy your appetite.

How is this beneficial for women? While Majority of the women out there and already tired and fed-up from stupid and lame dieting which hasn't worked out for them. And they have ended up gaining the lost weight in no time. Those women are done following any strict eating schedules and diet plans and are thus looking for some natural ways to lose weight.

This way of intermittent fasting brings ease to them, because they do not have to put any extra efforts or follow strict eating schedules.

They just have to slowly pace their appetite and move towards shorter portions of the meal. This will automatically bring the body in the habit of eating less and moving more thus enabling you to lose extra pounds without struggling.

Advantages:

- Convenient and simple.
- Slower than other techniques yet more beneficial.
- Losing weight without extreme dieting and exercising.
- Less calorie intake, higher possibility of weight loss.

How to get started with intermittent fasting?

Since now you have the information about what are the different ways and strategies for intermittent fasting, all you have to do now is to choose one method and implement it. The easiest way to get started is to pick a method that sounds easy to you and you think you will be able to pull-off. Begin it from there; see how it affects your overall health and energy. It is true that in the start you will feel a little weak but observe for longer patterns, if you do re-gain your energy levels even after implementing the fasting then keep on going. If the method is not suiting you or your body in any way, then you can stop and move on towards another strategy.

Intermittent fasting has a *learning curve* attached to it. It will take you some time to get habitual and understand what your body is telling you. You might not get it on the first try; you might have to browse through different ways and techniques of intermittent fasting to get it right. Keep on implementing the strategies until you find the best suitable fasting schedule.

Also, you don't necessarily have to follow a well-structured plan for intermittent fasting. As discussed before, there are some Intermittent Fasting strategies that don't require any strict schedule-following or calorie-counting. If you are a busy person and don't have much time to focus on the details then simply go for spontaneous fasting or random fasting days.

Even the strategy of making your meals small might do the job for you. It just needs some time to familiarize yourself with Intermittent Fasting and how it works.

In conclusion, if you are looking for pointers on how to start with intermittent fasting, you can go-ahead and read the 7-day beginner's guide for intermittent fasting. It has all the possible help and tips listed and you will not need much guidance after reading it. It has taken into account every possible consideration for beginners and has been made easy so that everyone feels welcomed and comfortable in beginning with intermittent fasting lifestyle.

Chapter 3

Design your own IF program

Intermittent fasting offers many programs and it is still possible that you don't find any of the described programs suitable for you. Fortunately, Intermittent Fasting extends the facility and ease of designing your very own program. You can choose your own day to fast as well as your own feeding and fasting window and you might be wanting to have just a few exceptions in your Intermittent Fasting program.

Must Note!

Designing your own Intermittent Fasting program is not recommended for beginners. You must first try some authentic Intermittent Fasting programs and experiment with them before moving on to defining your own. If you don't have any experience with Intermittent Fasting before, then while creating your own program you may go wrong somewhere and might also make mistakes which may impact your health and body. So initially, follow a recognized Intermittent Fasting program, follow its directions and then after experimentation with different Intermittent Fasting programs you find none of them are suitable for you, you can move on to designing one of your own. That way, you will have some helpful pointers and experience that will guide you how to get the best out of intermittent fasting.

Helpful pointers for designing your own IF program: You will notice that all the Intermittent Fasting programs have a few common things. These commonalities can act as your reference guide and can provide you a general guideline on how to design your own Intermittent Fasting program. Few of the commonalities are listed below for your ease:

- Fasting period is generally longer than feeding period.
- All IF programs have a 'feeding state' and a 'fed state'.

- In none of the programs the fasting window exceeds 24 hours. So, make sure, do not design a fasted state comprising of more than 24 hours because in that case it will be called 'starvation' and not 'fasting'.

How to design your own IF program? Researches have shown that many women frequently ask questions about how to design a successful Intermittent Fasting program, what things to include and what things to avoid. So, here is a general explanation of the guidelines that you should follow in order to design a completely healthy and successful IF program.

1) *Decide how often would you like to fast?* Would you prefer it doing daily, weekly or every other day? This decision is solely based on your work schedule, your lifestyle and your will to lose weight. If you want great results and you are very serious for losing weight then you might lean towards daily fasting. It is slightly hard, but very efficient. And if you are just casually exploring different types of fasting and do not want to lose too much too fast then you may incline towards weekly schedule where you just need to fast one or two days a week. So, first of all decide how often you would like to fast depending on your preferences.

2) *Decide how long can you fast?* If you are just entering the intermittent fasting world, then you should choose shorter fasting periods. But if you have a few months experience with Intermittent Fasting, then you can opt for longer periods of fasting. This all depends on your stamina, your willpower and your health condition. People with higher stamina and better health can go for long fasts, but people with low stamina and already low energy levels should try short fasts. Spontaneous fasts can also help you in this regard. Thus, decide how long you can fast and it should not exceed 24 hours!

3) *Decide what you want to eat during your feeding window?* Are you thinking why this is important? It is important because if you just had a sandwich in your feeding window, then it is likely that you will get hungry again much faster and thus your next fasting window will have to be short. But if you had a big and healthy meal after your fast, then you can go for longer duration of fasting the next time. Remember that eating healthy during your feeding state is important and your body will benefit from it. It might even heal your body and provide strengthening nutrition to your body.

4) *Put your plan in execution phase!* Now that you have figured out what to do and when to do it, you can now put your plan in action. It is better if you start out your Intermittent Fasting program the very next day or week depending on which type of Intermittent Fasting you chose. If you keep on delaying it onto next day or next week, you will never be able to start. Do it and do it now! If you keep on postponing it, an anxiety will keep on building inside your mind and that anxiety might lead you towards fear of starting. Plan well and start immediately. This will spare you all the drama and anxiety and might even help you to feel enthusiastic towards this experience.

Protocols necessary to succeed in intermittent fasting

Although Intermittent Fasting is itself a well-rounded technique and doesn't require extreme measures to be taken to succeed. Still, there are some factors that contribute in its success factors and some protocols need to be followed to get the best possible results in a shorter time. You can adjust the eating and fasting windows; you can choose the fasting days according to your will but there are a few necessary guidelines you need to know. Listed below are some important protocols to keep in mind in order to achieve 100% success rate through Intermittent Fasting:

Food quality. One of the most important factors that contribute in the success of Intermittent Fasting is the food quality. If you have been fasting and then you satisfy your appetite by junk food or unhealthy food every time; your body will not receive the necessary nutrients and proteins. This will leave a negative impact on your body; more importantly on your health. Intermittent Fasting doesn't restrict you to specific foods but it does recommend to eat healthy. Intermittent Fasting doesn't prohibit you from eating what you like but it does require a balance in diet. If you had a burger or pizza for lunch, have something healthy for dinner. The quality of the food matters too. Don't keep eating old food. Have a fresh meal every time. This will help you feel healthier and more energized.

Consistency. Second but important factor is *'Consistency'*. Just like all other dieting plans, Intermittent Fasting also requires its practitioner to be consistent. You might not get best results soon, but remain consistent and keep following the strategy for longer periods of time in order for it to work. It's possible that at first, you might feel the urge to quit, but research shows that women who stuck with it for extended periods of time were the ones happiest from its results. So, after you pick out an intermittent fasting strategy or schedule, stick with it and hold on to it and don't lose consistency.

It's a famous quote that 'good things take time' and it is 100% true while following intermittent fasting. Never lose hope or get disappointed if you don't see results instantly. Just believe and keep going on until you hit your goal-weight.

Calories. It is true that Intermittent Fasting doesn't put extremely harsh restriction on calorie count; still the calories do matter. If you fast for some hours and then relish a heavy meal with thousands of calories, you didn't do yourself any favors. Eating "normally" is the key here.

This means that when you are in the non-fasting phase; don't try to make up for the lost calories by eating huge meals. Eat normally as you would even if you hadn't been fasting. Some people believe that since they stayed hungry for a longer duration, high calorie intake won't affect them since they lost so much already.

It is not at all true. Yes, you have lost a good number of calories when you were fasting, but it does not mean you can eat more than you need or more than your appetite. Maintain a balanced diet regardless of the fact that you were fasting or not. This will help you lose more calories and gain less.

Patience. Studies have shown that many impatient people tried Intermittent Fasting and gave it up after a few weeks or a month. Just because they didn't see distinguished results in a short time, they decided to leave the practice altogether. This is not right. Once you get into something; be patient and wait for it to work, especially when you are guaranteed that you will see the results. It can take longer than you thought. Just be patient and keep giving complete dedication to it. It is also a fact that Intermittent Fasting takes longer than any of the crash-diets or extreme dieting plans. But it is also true that Intermittent Fasting takes a more natural approach towards losing weight. Diets might give you results sooner than Intermittent Fasting, but be assured that you must have left some nutritional deficiencies in your body that you might not be able to catch-up later. In the long run, diets have put people to bed because it insinuates hundreds types of diseases. Intermittent Fasting on the other hand; works naturally, doesn't ask for drastic changes, doesn't limit you to specific foods and recommends you to eat everything in a healthy and proper amount. So, it might take longer than dieting plans, just be patient and keep following the instructions with complete faith and be rest assured that you will lose weight and make your body healthier.

Training. There can be two types of training protocols – strength training and general learning training.

- General learning training includes to familiarize with yourself how Intermittent Fasting works, what are different strategies to implement and learning which implementation strategy works best for you. Since you have to test out different techniques and it has a learning curve attached to it; that is why it is called general learning training.
- Strength training means training your body to lose most of your body fat while holding onto muscle weight. Women who are at a healthy weight already and they just want to stay at their goal weight without losing muscle mass lean towards this training. In order to not get extremely skinny and look slim; strength training is provided. In this training you learn to keep on your muscle mass and just lose the extra fats and calories. This is very important regarding the health of your body because you never want to go overboard with fasting and become extremely weak. A good shape of body needs muscle mass and muscle strength, and in order to maintain a good and appealing shape of the body, understanding and implementing strength training is important.

Significance of fluids during intermittent fasting

Fasting windows doesn't allow any food intake, but researches have proven that drinking water and non-sugary fluids speeds along the process of weight loss from fasting. Keep yourself hydrated and use calorie-free drinks for the purpose.

You can drink as much water as you want, both normal and sparkling, unsweetened tea, lemon water and black coffee, because during intermittent fasting, water is the best choice. But if you are not in the mood of plain water, just add a simple mint or lemon for flavor.

You are allowed to have coffee and unsweetened tea also, but remember nothing works as best as water.

Why is water important? Drinking plenty of water is not only beneficial for keeping your body hydrated but there are many other numerous health benefits too. One, water carries oxygen and other healthy nutrients and leads them to your body cells, which helps in strengthening of the body cells.

Second, it helps maintain a healthy blood pressure. Third, it keeps your body temperature regular. Fourth, it keeps your digestive system healthy and regular. Fifth, it keeps your joints lubricated and strengthened. Therefore, during fasting when you are denying food from your body, it is necessary to provide nourishment to your body by drinking plenty of water. Some people don't realize its significance and its vital role in your health and that water deficiency later takes on a horrific shape for you in the form of a chronic disease.

What else can you drink?

- *Black coffee* doesn't take you out of your fasting cycle. And many published reports imply that caffeine can boost your metabolism and this also plays a role in losing weight. But it must remain simple black coffee; any added sweeteners or cream/milk can take you right out of your fasting cycle.
- *Tea* that is free from added sugars is also beneficial during intermittent fasting. It not only helps in cellular detoxification but also induces probiotic balance.

Although you can have all types of tea during your fast like green, black or herbal. But **green tea** specifically has proven to be more advantageous than other forms. It suppresses the levels of appetite and also it speeds the process of weight loss.

- *Apple cider vinegar* can also be kept under use during an intermittent fast. It helps in regulation of your blood sugar and also improves digestion. That's why it might enhance the effects of intermittent fasting.

Drinks to avoid during Intermittent Fasting. Many zero-calorie beverages are available in the market, which are actually full of calories. And intentionally or unintentionally, such beverages can put you out of your fasting cycle and can knock your body out of the fasted state. Such drinks include diet soda, coconut water, sugar-free juices, alcohol and almond milk.

Diet sodas claim that they are technically free of any calories, but it is all untrue. The artificial sweeteners added are worse than normal soda because they spike-up your insulin levels and also wreck your blood sugar levels. Also, coconut water and almond milk might sound like they are free of sugar but they are not. In fact, consuming these will increase your carb intake and you will eventually be put out of your fasted state. Same goes for alcohol.

Why avoiding sugary drinks is important during IF? Drinking sugary beverages initially spike your blood sugar, after that your body goes through a dramatic drop of sugar level and this prompts your body to eat more to bring back your sugar levels to normal. As a result, you are unable to withstand fasting since your body needs to regain sugar levels. And that's how majority of people lose their fast cycle and immediately are out of intermittent fasting. High sugar levels also prove to be addictive to your body and that's why you feel a craving again and again in your brain. Once you have a sugary beverage, next time when you fast your body will go in a low sugar level state and it will intensely demand from you the sugar-high that you gained from the sugary beverage. This will make it harder for you to resist eating, might even annoy you and might create a bad impression of fasting.

Take-away. Healthy beverages like water help you to overcome some common fasting concerns. It helps in curing headaches, dizziness, constipation and also muscle cramps. Hence, drinking plenty of fluids during fasting is extremely important. Also, consuming sugar-free and carbs-free fluids will help you maintain a healthy fasting cycle and as a result you will lose weight much faster and more efficiently. Beware of market claimed sugar-free products and always remember, any product that claims to be sugar-free must do something to make the taste good. That can sometime include artificial flavors, unnatural sweeteners or even some chemicals. Therefore, always tend to go towards natural and healthy beverages like water.

Helpful tips for intermittent fasting

Always start out slow. Before starting any diet or exercise or even fasting, always begin from the lowest level. Initially, you know that you are putting your body to go through a change and your body isn't prepared for it. Human bodies adapt and change with time and practice. You cannot expect that you fasted one day and the very next time you fast your body will be get into a habit of fasting. NO! Each body takes its own time to adjust and adapt to new changes and challenges put in front of it. Intermittent fasting offers beginner level as well as advanced levels. Beginner levels include the 8-hour eating window method and reducing meal portions.

Advanced levels include alternate day fasting in which you fast straight for 24 hours and alternate the days of fasting. It is mere stupidity to start from advanced levels. This will create thousands of deficiencies in your body because you didn't give time to the body to adjust to new changes and might end up with a chronic disease one day due to un-fulfillment of necessary nutrition.

Therefore, start from easiest level and progress your way to the top. Allow your body to adjust to new changes and focus on keeping a healthy nutrition

Experiment and learn. Intermittent fasting demands a certain level of experimentation from its practitioners. Some women might think that they can start-off with daily intermittent fasting but as they start, they begin to realize it is getting tough from them. Now this was an experiment that didn't give them the best results or didn't prove what they hoped for. What they should do is; to start spontaneous fasting. This will prepare the body to be more ready when and if you fast. So, you performed an experiment, deduced the results and learnt what technique is best for you and what strategy suits you the best. That is why; intermittent fasting is called experiment and learning technique.

Listen to your body. Human bodies are designed to adjust with new changes and with the passage of time get adapted to the changes and become habitual of them. Human bodies are embedded with the ability to send out warning signals to the brain if something is getting too much exhausting and tough for the body. For example, people under chronic stress begin to have constant headaches. The headaches are a sign from the body that the stress you are going through is too much for your body and you need to relax and calm your nerves. Similarly, when you start with Intermittent Fasting, the body initially will give you signals of weakness or even dizziness.

These initial symptoms happen and there is nothing to worry about. Just give time to your body to adjust. Intermittent Fasting demands time, and if after several months of fasting, still your body is giving signals of fatigue and low energy, it means that you are doing too much or your body is unable to cope with the loss of energy. It is also possible that after you have started intermittent fasting, in a month or so your body gets completely adapted and used to the new eating schedule.

Therefore, after passing the initial stages of fasting, keep an ear on what your body is telling you. If you feel fit and healthy even after fasting that means your body is in a healthy condition. But if you keep feeling dizziness or laziness, this might be a signal from your body that it's getting too much. Remember to always listen to what your body is telling you.

Slow and steady wins the race. Start-off at the beginner level and progress your way to harder and advanced levels of intermittent fasting. It works best, if you keep moving slowly and steadily. Do not act rashly and jump towards hardest levels of Intermittent Fasting. This will snatch away the adjusting and coping period from your body and this will leave you with hundred kinds of nutritional deficiencies or even some kind of diseases. Pick an intermittent fasting schedule, stick to it for months and then see the results and decide if the schedule has worked out for you. Don't expect extremely fast results. Intermittent Fasting is a natural way to reduce weight and that is the reason why you need to go slowly and steadily and remain consistent.

Write a journal or a make chart about your progress. Writing a journal or making a chart will help you track your progress and will help you in remembering what problems you faced. You can start from entering your initial weight and then after every week or every month, you can update it with your current weight and mention the weight-loss. Start by making a column called first week and enter all the information related to your first week in intermittent fasting. If you faced any dizziness or light-headedness, mention it down and see after how long these signs vanish.

If they vanish after a week or 10 days then be satisfied and know that you are on the right track. If they don't go away, it means that your body is trying to tell you something. If you keep on recording the intensity of these signs, it will help you to diagnose what is the root cause of this problem.

You can also write about your daily food experience. One day if you enjoy a slightly heavier meal and the next day you just eat some veggies, then it will be beneficial for you to compare the results and see which day you felt better. If heavy meals made you feel lazy and less energetic then you can have helpful pointers on how to avoid it from happening again. You can track the patterns of eating; see how different foods affect your health and activity of the day. At the end of the day, you can decide for yourself if you are progressing or if intermittent fasting is not suitable for you.

Be more active and productive. This It is a common perception that when you are fasting, you should rest and not move around much since your body is going through fasting window. This perception is not healthy and doesn't work out for the best. Remember, always act "normal"; doesn't matter if you are fasting or not.

"Acting normal" means continue to be active throughout the day, eat in the same way if you weren't having been fasting and this is the way to precisely train the body to get used to new Intermittent Fasting schedule.

If you think that after fasting and getting plenty of rest and eating a heavy meal afterwards is necessary to make-up for lost energy then you couldn't have been more wrong. The main purpose of Intermittent Fasting is to enable individuals to fast and lose weight naturally.

That means continue with daily jobs and activities as if you are not fasting. Staying active and productive will keep your body in a healthy and active state and will keep you energized throughout the day.

During the eating windows; choose nutritious foods. After completing the 'fasted window' when you enter the 'feeding window', always keep in mind to eat as if you were not on a fast and it is just another normal meal of the day. Also, your body needs necessary nutrients like protein and iron, so you must include healthy items on your menu. This will help restore the nutrition of the body and will keep you energized enough for further fast days.

If you relish an unhealthy and heavy meal after a fast, it will slow down your metabolism and create tons of digestive problems. So, maintaining a healthy diet is very crucial for the success of intermittent fasting.

Eat everything but in small portions. The best thing about intermittent fasting is that it does not limit your food choices.

Unlike diets, which limit you to only few foods, Intermittent Fasting doesn't restrict you in this regard. You can eat anything you wish to eat. The only condition is to maintain a balance. That is, if you ate heavy meal at one time then you should eat something very light and healthy in the next meal. Don't restrict what you eat, just limit everything you eat. Eating relatively smaller portions of meals each day will automatically train your digestive system and metabolism to stay active and work at their best at the given conditions. Thus, you will not be forced to abstain from foods you love, every once in a while, you can have whatever you want to eat.

IF is a convenience; not a strict obligation. Dieting plans are designed to be strict and put limitations to your overall eating habits. Dieting forces you to keep eating one type of food; for example, low-calorie foods. Dieting restrict you to eat very less after huge intervals of starvation. There is no wiggling room according to each individual. There are strict rules that everyone has to follow. This is where intermittent fasting comes in.

If provides you a much convenient option than dieting. You can choose your own fasting schedule; you can choose whatever you want to eat and you also get to choose when to eat it.

Intermittent Fasting allows you to define your own fasted and fed states and this allows every individual to feel comfortable and convenient with this weight-loss method. Therefore; people who enjoy a restriction-free lifestyle and want to be in charge of their own eating habits, lean much more towards intermittent fasting rather than conventional dieting methods.

Intermittent Fasting provides a comfortable, convenient, flexible way for women who want to lose a weight while enjoying their life and keeping their bodies healthy.

How to use IF for muscle gain?

The most negative and the worst side-effect of dieting is that body burns muscle along with the fats. This side-effect takes a strong negative toll on your health. Instead of losing excess fats, you start to lose your muscle which makes you weak from inside. Dieting has strict calorie restrictions and after losing fat it induces the loss of muscle inside the body.

Many research studies have been conducted in this regard and it has been proven that intermittent fasting interestingly lets you hold on to muscle while burning fat. The researches have shown that dieting induces 25% reduction in muscle mass and this is catastrophic in the long term. That's why intermittent fasting is extremely beneficial for women who are trying to hold on to their muscle mass and just shed-off the extra pounds they have gained.

How to gain muscle during IF? If you are working out while fasting side by side, you are more likely to burn more fat while sustaining muscle. Insulin sensitivity is the relation between the two.

If you are decreasing your calorie intake during your feeding window then you will burn higher fat in your fasting window. This means that when you consume food it is distributed how it should be. It will take place of the lost energy and will leave your muscle mass alone. People are always looking to hear this good news that the food you eat serves the right purpose. So intermittent fasting gives this good news to the people who are looking to lose fat while keeping muscles intact. The quality of the food you consume during your 'feeding window' decides the muscle growth and weight loss. If you are constantly consuming low-quality foods then you will lose the strength of the muscles eventually.

Weight loss is a must when you fast, but if you want to gain muscle while doing so; you must increase the quality of the food you are eating. It should be healthy and nutritious so that weight-loss doesn't draw out muscle mass too.

Tips for gaining muscle during intermittent fasting:

- If you are looking to increase your muscle gain, then you don't need to worry about meal timings too much. Just keep fasting and feeding on a regular basis and you will see that you will lose weight while keeping your muscle mass intact.
- Don't be afraid from calorie-restrictions. After fasting, you can enjoy a healthy and moderate sized meal. You shouldn't worry about only eating low calorie foods and restricting your meal portions. Eat freely to satisfy your diet.
- Do not restrict yourself from different kinds of foods. Integrate all kinds of foods in your diet, because you never know what food helps you the most to lose weight while incessantly gaining muscle mass.
- Simply changing your meal timings can significantly promote muscle growth. When you only eat at restricted timings every day, you will only lose weight and it won't affect your muscle growth. So, keep on changing the time of your meals and see what timing best suits your muscle growth.

- When we fast our insulin, levels drop and it helps to burn the fat, when we eat our insulin levels increase and helps to restore the energy of the body. Therefore, keeping an abstaining attitude from calories will help you lose weight, but it won't help you in increasing your muscle growth. So, during your feeding window, don't feel restricted from what to eat and what not to eat. Eat freely and eat healthy.

Common mistakes to avoid during intermittent fasting

Many people start out with intermittent fasting with high hope, but because of some conscious or unconscious mistakes they have a bad experience with it. These mistakes might hinder in the way of effective weight-loss, overall satisfaction and ease of the process. Below listed are few of the most common mistakes that are observed way too many times. So, providing information about them and highlight the ways to avoid them is important.

Giving up too early. Any weight-loss program is hard. Either it is dieting or workout exercises or even intermittent fasting. You are keeping yourself in a fasting state and that means you have to avoid from eating food for several hours. This is not easy to do at first. Your body is in a habit of receiving continuous nutrition.

And then when you start to fast, you are stopping the nutrition supply. So of course, you are going to face difficulty in initial stages of fasting. You will experience feelings of exhaustion and irritability.

But be assured that these feelings will go away after a week or two. Just be patient and wait for these symptoms to go away.

Once your body gets used to the new schedules, you will feel much more energetic and healthier. And you will start to really appreciate intermittent fasting. The main point here is not to give up too early. Everything demands time. It is also quite possible that the fasting method you chose doesn't fit quite well with your lifestyle.

So, don't hurry and throw in the towel too soon. Just hold on patiently and experiment with different types of fasting methods and see what works best for you. Rashly deciding that fasting is not suitable for you and giving it up too quick is one of the biggest mistakes that people make. You must know that intermittent fasting needs you to be calm, steady and patient. Results of Intermittent Fasting also can take longer than any other dieting plans, but the wait will be worth it.

Making drastic changes in your eating patterns. Too much change too suddenly can have negative impacts instead of positive. If normally you eat after every 3 to 4 hours and then suddenly one day shrink the eating window of the entire day to an 8-hour window, then this might be too drastic change for your body. You will be left feeling discouraged and hungry all the time. This is one of the biggest reasons that make people quit fasting. Each body needs time to adjust to new changes and everyone has different adjusting time. The quote 'slow and steady wins the race' works best in this situation. If you suddenly start from a 14 or 16 hour fast, your body won't be able to catch-up to such drastic changes. It may take you a week or 10 days to adjust to new schedules and long fasting windows. Gradually stretch out the number of hours between each meal and once you reach a 10 or 12 hour gap between your meals, then start a regular and strict fasting schedule. Because then your body will be ready to take the challenge and you won't feel lethargic or exhausted. After this, move towards a 10-hour eating window and slowly progress towards 8-hour feeding window. This is the way to slowly teach your body how to deal with the changes induced by limited calorie intake.

Eating heavy meals after fasting. After fasting, when you are feeling hungry, it is normal to overeat, because our body was hungry.

But overeating and overloading on calories will kill the soul of fasting. This will flush down your entire day's effort and you won't be able to reap the benefits of fasting. Especially when you are trying to lose weight, if you take much more calories than you lost during the fast, then you won't lose any weight.

Because the number of calories you gained due to overeating exceeded the number of calories you lost during your fast. A simple equation must be remembered in order for successful weight loss and that is *number of calories lost should be greater than number of calories gained.*

Also, if you are following shorter fasting periods and lose less calories, but then balance them out after eating, that won't also help you lose weight which will in return create an impression in your mind that Intermittent Fasting doesn't work. Although, the blame of not losing weight goes on your extremely high calorie intake after fast, yet you still end up quitting the healthy lifestyle of intermittent fasting.

An easy solution to this problem is that when you sit down to eat after your fast, do not pile up your plate with food. Instead, divide your food intake into a number of meals. *A meal divided into several small portions is better than one huge meal.*

Another mistake people make is to eat fast when hungry. When you eat fast, you end up eating more than needed. Eating slowly will help you satisfy your appetite by eating less. It will give you a feeling of stomach-full after eating less. So, when you are trying to lose weight fast, avoid these eating mistakes and you will see best results in no time.

Eating unhealthy. Some people think that intermittent fasting is a magical technique that will resolve of all their problems on its own.

Yes, it is true that Intermittent Fasting is an incredibly effective tool that will not help you to lose weight but will also restore your health. Intermittent Fasting cannot work if you are consuming a diet full of processed foods and sugars so, when you are fasting, it becomes more important to nourish your body with healthy foods than before. During intermittent fasting, your body becomes much more dependent on the foods you eat.

So, Intermittent Fasting will work best of you eat healthy foods and won't work at all if you eat unhealthy foods. Intermittent fasting is not just about the number of calories you consume, its more about eating nutrient-dense foods. Suppose you consume 500 calories of fruit one day and the next day you consume 500 calories of fried potato chips.

The day you had 500 healthy calories gained from eating fruit, that day you will observe higher energy levels, an overall healthy feeling and higher stamina. In contrast, when you had 500 calories of fried foods, it will not only keep your body from receiving nourishment but will also make it harder for you to fast. Try and maintain a balance of all macronutrients like iron, fiber, healthy fats and carbs.

Your body needs all the possible nutrition since it is working hard to burn the excess fats from the body. So, don't make the rookie mistake of eating unhealthy foods and then claiming that intermittent fasting doesn't work. It works best when you incorporate healthy and nutritious foods in your diet and keep a healthy schedule of fasting and eating.

Not drinking enough water/fluids. This is the most disastrous mistake anyone can possibly make during intermittent fasting.

When your body is under fasted state, it starts to decompose the damaged components and detoxifies the body. It is extremely important to flush out those toxins from your body by drinking plenty of water and other fluids. Ideally, you should drink more when you are fasting. Absence of water won't allow the toxins to leave the body and thus will hurt your body rather than healing it.

During a fast, you miss out on the hydration that fruits and vegetables provide your body. Not drinking enough water will push your body into a state of dehydration. And you must note that dehydration leads to several hundred other problems like headaches, muscle cramps and many others. Sometimes you might feel intense hunger pangs during your fast and you might mistake them happening because you are hungry. Sometimes, these pangs are a sign that your body is in dire need of water.

So, make sure to drink plenty of water during fasting, this will keep your body satiated during fasted windows. Plus, you will avoid many health problems caused by dehydration.

Forcing your body. Intermittent fasting might not be the best option for every single human being. Each body is designed differently and it is quite possible that intermittent fasting doesn't work for you. It has been reported several times that some people complain that they didn't lose any weight even after months and months of struggle and it is ok to acknowledge it. Everything doesn't suit everyone. You do not need to go out of the way to force your body. Not each body is built for intermittent fasting.

If you are a woman that has a body type which carries extra fat all the time, then it is quite possible that your metabolism is slow.

Slow metabolism leads to late food digestion and this might not give enough time to your body to start burning fat during the fasted state. On the opposite, if you are a woman with very fast metabolism and digestion, then you might find fasting extremely difficult to implement. It is totally fine to listen to what your body is telling you and if it is telling you to stop and get it out of the misery then do so. You do not need to force and push your body to must follow intermittent fasting. In fact, forcing your body might produce even worse results and might perpetuate imbalance in your body. If intermittent fasting feels like a continuous struggle and you are not getting used to the fasting schedules, then you do not need to drain your mental health. Just take a step back, re-evaluate the best method for you to opt for weight-loss.

Choosing wrong Intermittent fasting strategy. The biggest reason why any diet fails is because of their extreme contrast without daily life habits. The intense schedules and strict calorie restrictions contrast hugely from their normal eating routine and that's why people often feel impossible to maintain such hardcore schedules.

Similarly, talking about intermittent fasting, if you are used to of eating after every hour or two, then adapting alternate day fasting or 8-hour eating window might feel impossible to you. Sometimes you may rush into this and choose the wrong fasting style.

If you don't have the potential of staying hungry then you should start from 12 or 14 hours of eating windows and slowly progress towards 8-hours feeding window method. Another easy way is to start by 12/12 method. This will allow you a 12 hour fasting window and a 12 hour eating window. You can further divide each 12 hour into a 6-6 hour strategy and this won't make you feel you are stepping into something extraordinarily tough. You have to work on fasting styles yourself and see what fits best for you. But choosing the wrong method of fasting and then giving up on the entire practice is not a wise thing to do. Don't set yourself up for misery by signing up to something you already know is going to hinder with your lifestyle. Everyone has a different nature and attitude towards eating schedules. If you are used to of staying awake at night, then don't plan to start your fast at 6 or 7 PM.

If you love to go to the gym every day, then don't choose a fasting plan that restricts your calorie consumption to few days a week. It is all dependent on you and your lifestyle; choose a fasting plan that you think you can do and can along with your lifestyle.

Take-away. YES, it is possible that you might make some of these mistakes along the way during intermittent fasting. But it doesn't mean that you should give up on the entire method and claim that you cannot lose weight through Intermittent Fasting.

Each body is designed differently, so instead of rushing towards the decision that Intermittent Fasting doesn't work for you, perform some experiments with Intermittent Fasting methods and you never know the next method you try may suit your body completely and you successfully lose the extra weight. It is not a *hit-and-try* method; in fact, it *is try-try again till you succeed method.* If you started with weekly intermittent fasting and even after months you cannot see a significant change then it means that you made a mistake in judgment. Your body is not facing a challenge in weekly fasting. You should up your game and go for daily fasting. All of this is totally dependent on your intuition and judgment. Making mistakes is fine, not learning from them is bad.

Precautionary measures for intermittent fasting

Overly restricting your calorie intake is not necessary. If you are in your initial days of intermittent fasting, you should start to slowly restrict your calorie intake so that your body can get used to less intake with time. But if you have been practicing intermittent fasting for a long time now and you can easily pull-off 8-hour feeding window method or daily intermittent fasting, then you don't need to worry about your calorie intake. The reason is that your body is going through a long fasting window and providing necessary nutrition is important. Keeping track of calorie intake and overly obsessing about it is totally unnecessary.

The key is to be consistent with the feeding and fasting schedules and if you are regularly following the schedule then calorie intake should be the least of your worries. Do keep a general track and balance of the foods you consume, meaning if you had junk food for one meal then do balance it out with a healthy meal afterwards.

Making your meal portion smaller with time is a good practice for intermittent fasting and can help you in many ways. But over-doing can create deficiencies in your body. If you feel like you are hungry even after a small meal then enjoying a healthy snack afterwards can never hurt you. It's just that your body is telling you it needs more food and it is common to feel after a long fast. Thus, don't overly restrict your calorie intake, there is no hard and fast rule on the calorie intake in intermittent fasting and it's healthy to keep it that way.

Don't overdo it or go over-board. Some people are more eager than others to lose weight and integrate different intermittent fasting methods for a better and faster result. Because of their eagerness, they might go over-board with the fasting and it can turn out to be too much for their bodies. Women are already sensitive to the levels of insulin and if a slow and regular approach is not adopted, they might end up exhausting themselves too fast.

If you started with a 12 hour window of eating and fasting, then you might feel pretty confident about the fact that you can easily fast without any problem for longer durations. After that if you directly jump to an 8-hour feeding window, it might extremely difficult for you to manage the hunger levels. A 12 hour window is not very different from your normal routine, so keep in mind that progressing consistently though slowly is more beneficial rather than getting excited and putting your body through too much and end up going over-board. This will exhaust you faster and you will lose interest in the entire method just because of over-doing it.

Beware of what fluids to consume during 'fasting window'. As discussed earlier, many fluids and beverages out there in the market wearing a label of *sugar-free* are actually not sugar-free at all. They do add some artificial flavors or sweeteners instead of sugar to make it taste good. Beware of such drinks! They can take you right out of the fasting cycle and can also spike up your insulin and sugar levels in the body. Always go for water, sparkling or mineral or lime. You can also drink black coffee and various types of unsweetened tea. Consumption of fluids is although very important during fasting intervals but you have to be precautious about the nature of the drinks. A sugary drink will leave you with an instant sugar-high and then during your fast when your insulin level drops, you will suddenly crave those sugary drinks.

This makes it much harder for a person to fast for longer periods. Keeping your body hydrated during the fasting window carries vital significance for the health of your body. If you keep following the fast and feeding window properly and manage to fast for longer periods but forget to keep your fluid intake high; then your entire struggle can go down the drain. Intermittent fasting burns your fat and decomposes it into toxins, and in order to get rid of those harmful toxins, you need to flush them out by drinking lots and lots of fluids.

Never underestimate the power of drinking water during a fast. It will keep you satiated during the fast as well as it will get rid of the harmful side-effects of dehydration.

Focus on 'when' rather than 'what'. Intermittent fasting puts emphasis on eating schedule meaning 'when' and does not give much focus on 'what' to eat. Eating schedules, fasting and feeding windows carry more importance than what foods to eat to eat after fasting. If you focus on what to eat then you might neglect the importance of following fasting schedules. A balanced diet is although important in intermittent fasting but when you are talking about losing weight, calorie intake doesn't matter much. What matters is that you fast and enable your body to enter into the *fat-burning* mode. In order to lose weight, it is obvious that you have to get rid of the existing fat inside your body. And to that, your body needs to learn that when your insulin levels are low, that is you are under fasting state, the body needs to burn existing fat present inside your fat cells. This helps the process of calorie burning and thus acts as a pioneer for weight-loss.

Therefore, as a precautionary measure, stop worrying and fussing about calorie intake, what foods to avoid and foods to eat and solely focus on your fasting windows. Longer the fasting window, higher the fat burn, more the weight-loss.

Don't be hesitant in 'eating enough' during your feeding window. Eating enough and over-eating are two very different things. Eating enough means enjoying an amount of meal that sufficiently satiates your hunger and satisfies your appetite. Over-eating means to eat more than the demand of your body.

Intermittent fasting doesn't place any bounds what foods to eat, but just like any other weight-loss program, over-eating doesn't prove beneficial here as well. On the other hand, eating less than your appetite might also not prove healthy for some people. When you are not feeling full and want to eat more, it means that your body is in need of more nutrition. And to maintain a healthy body and a healthy lifestyle, you need to fulfill the nutrition requirements of your body. So never feel hesitant in satisfying your appetite. Eat enough but don't over-eat.

Female hormonal balance and intermittent fasting

Intermittent fasting affects women differently than men and there are several plausible reasons for it. Women have high sensitivity to hormonal changes. Female bodies trigger hunger hormones faster than a man's body when under the state called *fasted state* or *underfed state.* It is important for women to know that their bodies are not as much tougher like men's bodies, and they should treat their bodies accordingly. It is possible that a male member of your family is practicing a 24 hour intermittent fasting schedule and does not feel even a little weak or low on energy.

But if you try this schedule, it gets too much for you. This is normal and there is nothing to worry about here. There are many hormones inside a woman's body that get triggered way faster than men's. That's why there are more considerations for women than men related to intermittent fasting.

There are a few factors that induce hormonal imbalance in women and those are:

- Extreme stress (physical or mental)
- Not enough sleep
- Exercising way too much
- Not eating enough
- Not eating healthy

These are some of the reasons why your body might be under a hormonal imbalance. Intermittent fasting is known to improve metabolic rates and restore hormonal balance. If you follow Intermittent Fasting correctly and avoid the above-mentioned conditions, you will not only lose weight but you will also heal and nourish your body.

Intermittent Fasting allows you to start out slow, don't 'shock' your hormones by extreme starvation and maintain a healthy eating pattern. Regular eating intervals and healthier diet will help your body to fight with such imbalances. And intermittent fasting offers best eating patterns to its practitioners.

How does IF affect women differently than men?

Women tend to implement various ways for fast weight loss like exercising, workouts, different kinds of dieting etc. All the above mentioned ways are artificial weight loss techniques because you are not losing weight naturally. In fact, you are putting your body through a lot of pressure to shed-off the extra pounds. Intermittent fasting has proven the most effective and beneficial technique for women. It takes a natural way to lose weight and does not create any nutrition deficiencies.

Women need higher nutrition than men and are more sensitive to signs of starvation. They need all sorts of vitamins and minerals to keep a healthy body. They have the responsibility of managing the entire household, take care of their family, juggle work and also give birth to a new person. So, strict dieting and cutting-off nutrition can seriously harm the health of a woman. It might induce hormonal imbalance, hundreds of deficiencies and weaknesses.

Therefore, IF brings a safe and easy way for all the women out there to safely achieve their goal weight without stressing their bodies and without removing necessary nutrients from their life.

Note! Extreme calorie restriction can hinder with female hormones and can cause problems like hormonal imbalance, infertility and irregular periods. This is why it's important that women who are intermittently fasting are not doing it to restrict their calorie intake, they should opt this for better health and wellness aspects.

Reason is that when extreme restrictions are induced on calorie intake, it slows down the metabolism and hinders with digestive system. It's possible that it might make your digestive system slow too and this will put your hormones out of balance and won't allow your body to function at most optimal levels.

Ask yourself and your body, Extreme or Moderate? Means that if your body tells you that you are pushing it way too much or forcing it too much then it means you are on extreme levels of calorie restriction.

And if your body feels well and fine during a fast because you eat healthy afterwards, it means that it's under a moderate state of calorie intake. Intermittent Fasting boosts energy levels, increases stamina, increases motivation and it also improves cognitive functions.

Women need higher energy levels and strict dieting will drastically decrease these levels. A slow and steady approach to limit the food intake is the best and safest approach here. Intermittent Fasting defines specific eating windows and complements a healthy diet and lifestyle.

Chapter 4

When should women avoid intermittent fasting?

There are times when women should avoid any diet plans or even intermittent fasting. This includes:

- Pregnancy
- Nursing
- Under chronic stress
- Having a history of eating disorders
- Having irregular sleep pattern

How IF helps women? Women's bodies are designed in such a way that it maintains prime fertility conditions so that they don't have to face fertility problems later. And this is a main reason why female hormones are much active and more sensitive than male hormones. It has been revealed through studies that starvation and stress when mix together, they can negatively affect the fertility of a woman. This means that if a woman is following extreme dieting plans and long starvation hours plus she is facing constant stress, then she may be hurting her own health.

Intermittent fasting is advantageous for women in this regard because unlike diets, women can choose however long they want to fast, depending upon their stamina and energy. If you are a working woman and several days of the week you work too hard or remain under stress, then you can easily opt not to fast on those days. Just simply choose the days of the week in which you have low work pressure and lower stress. You can do this through "weekly intermittent fasting" schedule and just choose 2 days of the week that you can easily carry a fast. Unlike diet programs; intermittent fasting actually cares about your health; both mental and physical. Intermittent Fasting creates a healthy eating schedule which simplifies your life thus reducing mental pressure. It also makes you follow a healthy diet plan which helps you to stay more active and productive. This increases your physical health.

Diets will leave your body all lazy and weak and they can also trigger hormonal imbalance.

Pros and cons of IF for women

Must Note! *Cons can only occur if you overly restrict your calorie intake, eat unhealthy, go past the limits of fasting windows and fast more than 24 hours.*

Pros	Cons
Sustainable weight loss	Disturbed metabolism
Increase in muscle mass	Irregular periods
Higher energy levels	Fertility issues
Reduction in inflammation	Anxiety
Improved insulin sensitivity	Difficulty in sleeping
Reduced oxidative stress	Shrinking of ovaries
Boosts up cognitive functions	Hormonal imbalance

7-Day Intermittent Fasting guide for beginners

To help you kick-start your intermittent fasting journey, here is a simple and easy to follow 7-day guide. If you have never tried intermittent fasting before and you are just starting your journey, then here is a convenient 7-day plan laid out for you so that you have a fun, easy and good experience.

The tasks and the goals for each day are specifically provided so that you don't start off too rash or make any mistake. For your first week, you should slowly ease into intermittent fasting so that your body doesn't go into a shock state.

DAY 1:

Fasting Window	Feeding window
12 hours	12 hours

For very first day of the first week, you should start off by choosing a convenient fasting and feeding window. This 12 hour window is not very different from your daily life and it will not pressurize your body on the very first day. The main goal of this activity and beginner's guide is to highlight the fact that you should slowly ease into the journey of intermittent fasting. If you start off hard and don't give enough time to your body to adjust, then chances are that you will torment your own health and might put your hormones into a shocked state. Going too fast too soon, can create many imbalances like hormonal imbalance or metabolite imbalance.

12 hour fasting and 12 hour feeding window means that you only have to fast for half a day. In our normal routine, the gaps between our meals add up to almost 12 hours and this doesn't differentiate much from our normal routine. Thus, this makes it easier for your brain and body to get used to and prepare for some eating changes. It will also give you more time to settle-in and adjust with the new fasting schedules.

Intermittent fasting though offers different kinds of programs for different people, but this guide will eventually put you with the *8-hour feeding window method.* That is, on Day 7, you will be starting with 8-hour feeding and 16-hour fasting window method. And you will continue with the most on following days.

Once you feel comfortable with this method, you can further shorten your feeding window and elongate your fasting cycle. It all depends on your body, if it allows you to stretch the cycles you can.

And if not, then keep following 8-hour method and with time you will see results that you have been looking for.

Goal of Day 1: For your day 1, you only have to *choose your intermittent fasting schedule.* Today's goal is very easy and very doable for you. You have to see, which fasting schedule best suits your lifestyle and routine and the schedule you want to follow after your initial training. The best thing is that for your first 7 days, you explore all fasting options while simultaneously putting your body in a habit of fasting slowly and steadily. After the 7 days complete, you can choose any intermittent fasting schedule; weekly, daily or even alternate fasting schedules. Stay consistent and keep following the 7-day guide and this will prove to be the most contributing factor to your success.

DAY 2:

Fasting Window	Feeding window
13 hours	11 hours

On day 2, your fasting window is extended to 13 hours. Just one hour more than yesterday. You can do it! Gradually increasing the window will allow your body to understand the new changes and will allow it to handle the new calorie intake. If you suddenly start-off with alternate day fasting which has a 2 hour feeding and fasting cycle, then your body will get confused on how to deal with such a big change in such a short time.

Now, you are getting familiar with how intermittent fasting works. Its might be possible that you don't feel much different than before which is a good sign. It means that your body is comfortable with the new fasting cycles. And if you are already feeling some low energy levels then there is nothing to worry about!

Usually all bodies take a 7 or 10 day time to adjust to this fasting schedule. That is why this guide is introduced so that you don't get afraid or anxious and quit Intermittent Fasting without giving it a worthy shot. Day 2 will introduce you to new healthy guidelines that support your goals of intermittent fasting. Guidelines will help you in losing weight and can also assist you in maintaining a healthier lifestyle.

Define your fasting goals and what you want to achieve by the end of the day. Either your goal is to just lose weight or if your goal is to learn and apply healthy eating schedules; simply focus on eating healthy and avoid the stress of counting calories.

Eat until you satisfy your appetite and remember not to overeat! Intermittent fasting cannot work until your body knows how to burn the fat inside the body. So, for that purpose, do not overeat. Eat just enough to satiate your appetite.

Goal of Day 2: Today's goal is to *learn the basics of intermittent fasting.* Learn about the importance of eating whole foods and avoiding processed foods and sugar. Learn about healthy carbs and empty carbs. Get to know about the significance of eating all types of healthy foods and provide all necessary nutrition to your body during the feeding window.

Think about what simple yet delicious meals you can prepare for yourself at home. Familiarize yourself with healthy fluids like water, black coffee and tea.

Avoid sugary drinks like juices, sodas and diet sodas. Learn about the benefits and advantages of keeping yourself hydrated during your fast and also get to know what happens if you let your body dehydrate.

Several hundred problems are born if you don't keep yourself hydrated, so make sure to drink plenty of fluids!

DAY 3:

Fasting Window	Feeding window
14 hours	10 hours

Day 3 is here with the increase of one more hour in the fasting window. Do not worry at all because you are totally capable of doing this! This guide is especially designed for beginners and it won't affect your health until you keep enjoying healthy meals. You are moving gradually and consistently and you should appreciate yourself for it. Each day, your body is getting stronger and stronger. With each day passing, you are adapting to a healthier lifestyle and better eating patterns.

Stay active and be productive. Don't let the concept fool you that since you are fasting you should reduce your activities and rest more. This won't help you. You have to get your body used to the fact that you will work just like you used to, the difference is that you are limiting your food intake to specific hours of the day.

Eating at better times will give your more energy to carry out your tasks of the day. Again, you might have some concerns if you are feeling tired and low on energy. Don't worry as there is nothing unusual going on. It is normal to feel a bit tired in the beginning of this journey and you have to give 4 to 6 more days to your body if you want to decide that either you want to continue or not.

Don't think of giving up earlier than 10 days. It usually takes 7 to 10 days for a human body to adjust to fasting. Believe that you can do it and know that you are not the first one fasting. Humans have been fasting since thousands of years now and their bodies are well capable to it. If they can, so can you! Just remain consistent.

Goal of Day 3: Today's goal is to *define your reward!* Defining your reward will keep you enthused and will inspire you to keep the hard work up. You can define reward for each day that you successfully fast or you can define a big reward when the 7 days end. Reward can be a simple cheering sentence like "Good job! You are doing great! Yes, you can do this!" or can be a bigger reward than this like a day out or a treat to go to a restaurant. Small rewards help you keep your spirits high and you remind yourself of what you can achieve. Saying these small sentences will help you to keep continuing until you achieve your goal weight. Bigger rewards are for people who find fasting difficult, they want to lose weight but they don't want to limit their eating habits. For such purpose, you can promise yourself something like 'if you lose a pound a week, you will get to treat yourself at a restaurant after that week'. These are just ways and tricks to keep yourself continue on the journey of intermittent fasting and one day reach your goal of weight or a healthier lifestyle.

DAY 4:

Fasting Window	Feeding window
15 hours	9 hours

Congratulations! You are more than halfway there. Today, you will be fasting for 15 hours already. The beauty of this technique is that it doesn't let you feel way out of routine and yet you are significantly progressing towards your goal each day. It's possible that you might already be seeing healthy effects of intermittent fasting schedule. You might feel you already have lost a little bit of weight but it is also normal not to feel a change just about now.

Be patient! Each body is designed differently and everyone has different metabolism rate. You don't need to worry if you have a slow or fast metabolism; just keep going on with this fasting schedule and your goal will not appear far away from you. If you are feeling extreme hunger pangs during your fast, it might be a signal that you are not eating healthy enough or you are drinking fewer fluids then needed. Remember; do not dehydrate yourself during your fast. Also beware of avoiding sugary fluids during your fast. Sugary fluids can break your fast and throw you out of the fasting cycle. We want a healthier body, not an even weaker body than before. And to deal with the problem of not eating enough healthy foods, today's goal is to have a very healthy meal rich in protein and nutrition.

Goal of Day 4: Today's goal is to *prepare a high protein meal.* Eating healthy and fulfilling your nutrition needs is necessary for success in intermittent fasting. So, today you are going to make yourself a protein-filled lunch. The protein can be of your choice like fish, grilled meat, eggs, beans or tofu. You can pair it up with steamed or grilled vegies and you will have a nutrition-dense meal in front of you. Women need all the possible nutrition during feeding cycle. So, in order to keep yourself healthy and active and in order to avoid nutrition problems, enjoy a healthy meal daily. Intermittent fasting doesn't restrict you on calorie intake. It also doesn't restrict you on what foods to eat. But eating healthy at least once a day during fasting days is very important in maintaining a good and healthy body.

DAY 5:

Fasting Window	Feeding window
16 hours	8 hours

You have successfully reached the 16/8 window goal. You will today be fasting for 16 hours with an 8-hour feeding window. Since you have been progressing slowly, today you won't feel it very hard to fast for 16 hours. But if you had started directly from 16 hour schedule, you would have been feeling very tired, exhausted and lazy. Following this guide has helped you to successfully reach your goal of fasting without putting your body through drastic changes.

Research has shown that hundreds of people have undertaken similar challenges. Some people have taken 21 day fasting challenge and some went for a shorter challenge. But the end results for all such challenges have been positive and satisfying.

These types of challenges also highlight the significance of taking it slow but they also challenge your body a little bit. Some people are satisfied with the results of these challenges while some are left behind because they have a slower pace than others and cannot keep-up with the challenge.

This 7-day guide is designed for all kinds of people. If you had no problem until now; then very well! Keep it up! But if you anytime feel that this is too much for your body then you can pause at whatever day you are and practice it for a few more days.

For example, if you are at day 3 where you have 14/10 window ratio and you felt that it was a little hard for you and you need more time to adjust, then there is nothing to worry about. Make day 4 also a 14/10 window and keep going until you are comfortable with it and then move on.

Goal of day 5: The goal for day 5 is *to drink fluids like green tea or black coffee if you feel hungry.* This will help you go through with 16 hour fast easily and will also curb your hunger. Also, keep in mind that water is the best fluid to drink during the fast. But if you want to curb your hunger a little bit you can drink these green tea or black coffee too. But don't overdo it! Black coffee is rich in antioxidants and also greatly helps to suppress the hunger. But you have to remember that you cannot add milk, cream or sugar to your coffee. This will increase your sugar and insulin levels and thus will be counted as eating. Similarly, if you want to drink tea instead of coffee, it is better to have green tea and it must be unsweetened. Sugar is a no-no in any case during your fast. So, sugar in any form should be avoided because it can instigate hunger.

DAY 6:

Fasting Window	Feeding window
16 hours	8 hours

Today you are staying with yesterday's schedule that is 16 hours fast and 8 hour feeding window. This right here is an intermittent fasting method and you do not need to go further if you don't want to. This is called 8-hour feeding window method and you can stick to it if you are comfortable with how things are right now.

If you are looking for a harder challenge then you should practice two more days; day 6 and day 7 with the same schedule and then move forward to something hard. Practicing the schedule, a little more will help you build your stamina for a much harder challenge and you will not face any difficulty once you move past this level. Just keep on going as you are, follow the schedule, keep eating healthy and be consistent no matter what!

Don't get overconfident and be too quick about it. If you didn't have any problem until now, it's good. But it doesn't mean that you are ready for anything to be put in front of you. Do not mess up everything by going too fast. You are in a great condition right now; follow this schedule for two more days and then move on to your decided intermittent fasting schedule. It is totally good and fine to stay here and practice as long as you want. Get used to it, no matter how much time it takes.

Goal for Day 6: The goal for the day is to *go for a walk*. If you already walk daily or you are already used of exercising a little bit daily, then it's great! Your job for the day is done. But if you haven't stayed much active during these fasting days, then start today.

It's your second day following 16/8 schedule, so don't worry about exhausting yourself. Your body knows that it has an 8 hour feeding window allowed and it will function optimally. Walking will also switch your focus from hunger and will help you pass the last hours of fasting much more conveniently. There is just a slight need of staying active and increasing the daily activity. The purpose is to build stamina in your body for physical activities during intermittent fasting. So, start-off by a small walk if you are not in a habit of it or walk as much you like if your body allows you.

Remember to listen to your body. When you feel tired, stop and go home. Tomorrow you will have a much higher stamina and you will probably walk double than today.

DAY 7:

Fasting Window	Feeding window
16 hours	8 hours

Today you keep your new 16/8 fasting schedule. While doing so, you will do some reflection on how your past week went. You will answer some common survey questions that people usually take at the end of this process. These questions will help you assess the overall experience. After you answer these questions to yourself, you will decide whether you want to continue with this schedule or do you want to shift to some other fasting schedule? The questions are as follows:

- How do you feel during and after your fast?
- Do you feel tired or fatigued?
- Is there any change in your energy levels?

- How was the experience? Did you enjoy it or was it a torture for you?
- Have you noticed any change in your overall mood?
- How is your skin's condition? Is it better than before or does it feel dry?
- What was your biggest struggle?
- Is there any change that you would like to implement?
- Does this schedule suit your lifestyle?

Goal of Day 7: Today your goal is to *decide which schedule of intermittent fasting to follow?* You will answer the above mentioned questions and that will help you decide if you want to stick with the existing schedule or do you want a bigger challenge?

You will assess how well your last week went and was it even a challenge for you or not? If it didn't feel like much of a challenge then go for even shorter feeding cycles. But if it was too much to take then either elongate the feeding window or move towards a weekly fasting schedule. Feel free to say out loud whatever you are thinking. There is nothing to be ashamed of.

Thousands of people decide that this is too much and they need to go towards a lighter fasting schedule. They go for what their body tells them and after a year or so they happily report back with the great news that they achieved their goal weight and that they are very happy now. Thus, follow your gut, openly answer the questions and strategize your future plan. This will help you accelerate the decision making process and you will be able to make intermittent fasting a new sustainable habit.

Is exercise safe for women during IF?

It all depends upon your stamina. Generally, women who exercise during intermittent fasting have had no problems. In fact, they report that it keeps them active and helps to burn more fat and thus weight loss is pretty fast. Exercise can greatly help with fat-adaptation. Glycogen (the stored form of glucose in your liver and muscles that helps body when you are under a fast) gets depleted when you fast or sleep and further depletes when you exercise.

What's the benefit of this? **This will increase insulin sensitivity.**

That means that when you have a meal after a workout, it will be much efficiently utilized by the body since it kept burning fat during the entire time. A meal after a workout will be stored in the form of glycogen in muscles while some of it is utilized to get the energy of the body back up. Least amounts are stored as fats and it can prove extremely beneficial for you when your goal is to lose weight.

Our body follows a simple rule of *"Higher insulin levels, higher fat storage"* and vice versa. Therefore, keeping insulin levels low is very important when you are trying to lose weight and exercise is one of the best ways to do it. When insulin sensitivity is at a normal level, the food consumed will be utilized for full glycogen storage in muscles; it will also be used as glucose in the blood stream and thus has a higher chance to get stored in the form of fat.

A good workout can help you regulate and increase your insulin sensitivity.

How to lower insulin levels (How to increase insulin sensitivity)? There are few things that can help to increase insulin sensitivity and those are:

- Intermittent fasting
- Exercise
- Low carb diet
- Low calorie diet
- Foods that are nutrient-dense

Safety concerns of exercising during fasting: Although it sounds like that exercise is the best and fastest option to lose weight. But there are some precautions that need to be considered before jumping to a decision. Long fasts and long workouts might push your body to start breaking down the muscle to use protein as a fuel.

This can have a negative impact on your lean muscle mass. Women who like to have abdominal muscles or arm muscles should note that extreme deprivation from food and extreme hard workouts will eventually take a toll on your muscle mass. So, if you want to maintain your muscle mass but want to lose weight, then do exercise but remain at moderate level of exercising. Don't work out too hard and for too much long durations.

How to safely exercise while fasting? If your ultimate goal is to reduce body fat while maintaining your fitness level and muscle mass then you need to keep your body in the safe zone. Listed below are some tips to successfully achieve your goal while exercising:

1) **The duration and intensity should be low**
   When longer duration of exercising is paired up with long fasts, your body can enter into a state of calorie deficiency. And in order to refuel itself, it will start to burn protein and energy present in the muscles. If you push yourself too hard, you can end up feeling dizzy or even light-headed. When this happens, relax and take a step back. Because it is a clear sign that you are forcing your body too much. Keep the intensity of the workout low too. Extremely hard workouts can create energy deficiency in your body. Therefore, just keep the duration and intensity of the exercise at a low level.

2) **Stay hydrated and keep your electrolytes up**
   During fasting, you should increase your water intake no matter if you exercise or not. Dehydration can cause several problems like headaches and it can also slow down the metabolism. If you are exercising as well as fasting, make sure to focus on keeping yourself hydrated and

keeping your electrolytes up. Choose a good low-calorie hydration source and stick with it throughout the process. Avoid sports drinks because they are extremely high in sugar and your goal is to lower the insulin levels, not spike them up.

3) **Eat a meal closer to your workout**

    It is a misconception that you should not eat close to your workout session. Always prefer eating a meal after a workout because that will help your body to get the most out of the food. Having a meal shortly after exercise will help your muscles to regain the strength because it will provide glycogen to it. The chances of food getting stored as fat become very low because your body balances out its fuel needs and utilizes it properly.

4) **Listen to your body**

    The most important thing is to listen to your body. If you are feeling dizzy or light-headed then it is possible that you are having very low blood sugar levels. It is also a sign of dehydration. So, in such a case, go for a healthy drink and then have nutritious and well-balanced meal. After that, reanalyze your workout style. It might be possible that you are pushing your body way too hard and you need to take a step back and shift towards a relatively low intensity exercise.

Conclusion: Exercise does not suit everyone while fasting. It may or may not work out for you. Some people feel perfectly healthy and more active when they indulge in a light exercise with a fast while others may not feel comfortable with exercise at all.

If your workouts are getting weaker as a result of fasting; it might be a sign that your body needs more nutrition or you need to try some other intermittent fasting schedule. And if the rest of your fasting cycle is working great for you but when you exercise you feel exhausted, then you need to ease up on exercising or workout methods.

Remember, always move steadily and start with low intensity; either it is exercise or it is intermittent fasting. Knowing when to back-off is important when you are trying both intermittent fasting as well as exercising.

Chapter 5

Why is autophagy important for women?

What is Autophagy? Autophagy is a process in which the body cleans out the damaged cells and then generates new and healthier cells. It is like a self-preservation system through which the body itself locates and removes the dysfunctional cells or repairs them. Even healthy human bodies experience cell damaging. As a result of our metabolic processes, it is very natural that cells constantly become damaged. Sometimes, with increased stress, the damaged cells also radically increase. And that's why nature introduced autophagy in our bodies.

Autophagy helps the body to clear out damaged cells or cells that have no functional purpose in the body. Such non-functional cells keep lingering inside our bodies until they are cleared out. Clearing them out is very important, because if such damaged cells don't clear out from our bodies, we can become more susceptible towards diseases and illnesses.

Is autophagy good for health? Researchers have proven that autophagy acts as a survival mechanism for our bodies and it's a way for the body to protect itself. Studies have also shown that autophagy is important in "cleaning up of the body" and acts as a defense strategy against higher stress levels. So yes, it is definitely good for our bodies. It is a key in preventing various types of diseases like cancer, liver disease, diabetes, autoimmune diseases and infections.

Relation between autophagy and intermittent fasting: To induce autophagy, intermittent fasting plays a significantly important role. To say that intermittent fasting causes the autophagy process to start won't be wrong. Different schedules of intermittent fasting can induce autophagy in a body including daily intermittent fasting (with a few hours of eating window) or alternate intermittent fasting (where you fast for 24 hours and then can eat for the next 24 hours).

Another easier way to induce autophagy through Intermittent Fasting is to eat one or two meals a day with a solid gap between them and don't snack in between. Staying hungry between several intervals will initiate low insulin levels inside your body and that acts as a signal that now the body needs fuel and it can only get from inside a body. That's when it starts burning fat as well as clears out hazardous and damaged cells. *That's how intermittent fasting plays a role in healing and restoring health to a body.*

Benefits of Autophagy:

- Unnecessary and dysfunctional cells are disassembled and cleared out from the body.
- It helps to fight infectious diseases.
- It strengthens the immune system.
- Prevents cancer and various other neurodegenerative diseases.
- Provides the cells with molecular energy.
- Recycles damaged proteins and regulates functions of the cells.
- Protects the nervous system.
- Enhances growth of brain and nerve cells.
- Improves strength and cognitive functions of the brain.
- Protects against heart diseases and helps in the growth of heart cells.
- Provides stability of DNA
- Prevents any damage to healthy organs and body tissues
- Mechanism that has anti-aging benefits.

Importance of autophagy for women: It is quite normal for women to have hormonal imbalance. Sometimes it happens because of disturbed metabolism and sometimes you may never know the reason. In cast when you don't know the reason of the imbalance, autophagy can come in and greatly help you. It restores the balance of your hormonal cells and can also discard any harmful or dysfunctional cells. Thus, for restoring your hormonal imbalance or for regulation of disorders; autophagy can play an important role.

And in order to induce autophagy you need to intermittently fast.

Secondly, Breast cancer is the most common and fatal cancer in women worldwide. A study has shown that roughly over a million women are diagnosed with breast cancer in a year. Though with the advancement of medical field it is not considered fatal now.

Cancer development can be controlled through autophagy. It hinders the way of progression of cancer and removes the defective cells growth. Autophagy plays a very important role in stopping the initiation of such cancel cells and if they have initiated already then autophagy stops their progression and discards those harmful cells out of our body. So, it is proved that autophagy is vastly beneficial for women. But again, the question stands:

How to initiate autophagy inside the body? Autophagy needs the triggering of cells and nothing triggers the cells better than intermittent fasting. So, fasting does not only help in losing weight, it also helps to induce autophagy inside a body which gets rids of all dysfunctional cells from the body. Thus, leaves your body healthier and fitter than before. Sometimes, the health-care providers suggest intermittent fasting for overweight women because the excess weight is making them susceptible towards many diseases. The reason why the medical practitioner or the doctor might suggest intermittent fasting is because they want to strengthen your immune system to fight against diseases that might occur due to obesity. So, don't worry about the extra fat on your body, it can be easily gotten rid-off.

Start intermittent fasting with an easy to follow schedule, it will not only help you with the weight loss but it will also help you increase health by inducing autophagy in your body. While Intermittent Fasting gets rid of your excess fat, autophagy will automatically get rid of dangerous and dysfunctional cells from your body.

Keys to improve general health

1) Be active. Staying active has numerous advantages for physical as well as mental health. Physical activity has hundreds of benefits and all of them can never be listed here. The most important benefit of staying active is prevention from chronic diseases.

Researchers believe that staying physically active can prevent many illnesses and diseases while it also cures mental problems like anxiety, stress and even depression. A healthy body just demands a little bit of daily exercise or walking or playing a game outside. It does not demand extreme hardcore workouts from you.

When it comes to physical health, there is a rule that the longer the better. It means if you walk for longer periods or stay physically active for a long time, then it helps to build higher stamina in your body. Physical movement can also help with weight-loss. It is because when your body is physically active and under motion, the body is constantly burning extra calories and fats for energy.

Staying active helps to build higher energy levels and lowers the fat levels. If you stay put and don't move around much, then the calories you daily consume have no way to burn themselves. As a result, they keep on piling up and you keep on gaining weight.

Therefore, stay physically active. It will solve almost all your health problems.

2) Have a healthy diet. People underestimate the power of a healthy diet. Because of the fact that they are too busy with their lives, they don't have enough time to prepare a healthy and proper meal for themselves. Instead they go ahead and eat whatever is available to them. Crappy foods will not be able to provide your body any energy whatsoever. After eating, very soon you will feel you are hungry again and it's because they didn't have any nutrition value in them. If you have a busy work schedule, it is more of a reason to eat to healthy. Eating unhealthy can put the female hormonal balance into a state of chaos. Female bodies need a much more nutritious supply of food than men. It's because of the fact that female bodies are designed to keep themselves running at optimal conditions so that they can go through childbirth and breastfeeding successfully. If your body doesn't receive nutrition enough for itself, how can it help you to have a healthy baby? Include everything in your meal including iron, protein, healthy fats and carbs. Don't restrict yourself to low-carb diet plans because this won't allow your body to receive complete nutrition which it is supposed to. Healthy eating, healthy lifestyle!

3) Maintain a healthy body weight. Healthy body weight is defined by body mass index (BMI) and it ranges between 18 and 24 if you going for normal BMI. With the advancement of science, there have been many studies conducted and there are several ways to calculate your BMI. The easiest way to do it is from online BMI calculators. You can find many online BMI calculators that ask you your height and weight in lbs. and it tells you your BMI and it also tells you if it is healthy or not. If it is in healthy range it will tell you that you have a normal BMI. If it is too high or too low, it will tell you that you have an unhealthy or abnormal BMI and you need to make efforts for a healthy and normal BMI.

Don't always focus on dieting and losing fats. Your body needs some energy sources, so better keep it that way. A few extra pounds won't hurt you until and unless you are maintaining a healthy diet. Although, if you are not eating healthy or at regular times, then your body weight gain may be a symbol of something else. For the body to work optimally, it needs proper nutrition, healthy diet and a well-maintained eating schedule. This allows you to stay from hundreds of problems like eating disorders, sleeping unwell, being more disposed to the diseases. Therefore, keep your focus on eating healthy and maintaining a healthy body weight.

4) Enjoy light exercise daily. Daily exercise has proven to be beneficial for the human body and numerous studies have been conducted for it. Results showed that women who exercise daily; not extreme hardcore workouts, just some light exercise showed better metabolic rates, higher digestion rate and better ability to get rid of the excess fats. Staying active is always suggested by health-practitioners and doctors, because it helps the immune system to grow stronger and helps it to fight-off a number of diseases. It also helps to maintain a better physical as well as mental balance. If you are stressed out too much, go for a walk and it is guaranteed that it will calm your nerves by releasing toxins out of your body. Some women enjoy a healthy workout while some are not comfortable with exercising. Those who work out daily should remember not to overdo it overstretch it and keep the workout at a normal level. If you work out extremely hard daily then once you give it up, it will do more harm than good. And women who are not in a habit of daily physical exercise should start by talking baby steps. Go for a small walk today and gradually increase your walk time and pace. When you build up enough stamina, your body will itself tell you what to do next. Mobilization of stored fats is necessary when you are trying to lose weight. Just by cutting off your diet supply might not do the magic. But throw in a light daily exercise; you will see your dream weight coming.

5) Think positive and stop stressing out. Research shows a healthy positive attitude helps in building a healthier and stronger immune system and boosts overall health. Your body will believe whatever you think, so think positive and focus on positive aspects of things in life and your body will also stay happy and positive. People with extreme busy work schedules and hard lifestyle must do some positive thinking in a day; it will energize their body and keep them enthused. Stress is a very common mental disease observed in people these days. They don't eat healthy and keep stressing out, which plays a great hand in destroying the immune system, destroying the metabolic rate, increases the chances of heart problems and dysfunctions the digestive system. On top of that, it stresses out your brain and nerve cells and constantly keeps on making nerve cells damaged or even dysfunctional. Whenever you feel stressed, just stop for one moment, close your eyes and take a few deep breaths. Deep breaths help slow-down the heart rate.

People who have lower resting heart rates are usually in a better physical condition than those who have higher rates. You can also practice meditation and light exercise. Prolonged stress to the heart can induce many health problems like high blood pressure, depression and obesity.

6) Shift to 5 small meals instead of 3 big ones. What, when and how much you eat affects directly your metabolism and energy levels. Suppose that after a long day of hard work, you missed a meal and when you get home, you overeat because you feel so hungry. This overeating will affect you in so many ways that you can't even imagine. It will slow down your metabolism, it will make you feel lazy and lethargic and it will put your digestive system out of order.

Therefore, shift to a 5 meal schedule, where you enjoy 5 small meals in a day. This will save you from getting overweight, you will avoid cravings and it will help you to maintain your cool and balance. A smaller meal will eliminate the chances of overeating and thus helps you stay active. A huge meal will slow down your body and make you lazy, it is because your metabolism slows down and the body has to work really hard to digest the meal. That's why you feel exhausted even after having a meal and you wonder why it is happening. Whenever you get a chance, divide your meals further. If you were going to have fried vegetables with a piece of grilled meat, then divide it into two portions and finish it in two meals. Or enjoy the meat now and then eat vegetables later. This will keep your metabolic rate up and you will feel energetic after eating and not lazy. It will also help your body to get the most out of a meal and not just store it up in the form of fats.

7) Get a good night sleep. Sleeping disorders are commonly observed in people these days. If you are having trouble sleeping, you can always try peaceful techniques such as meditation and yoga. This will help you calm your nerve cells and will bring peace to a stressful mind. A reason why you might be going through a sleeping disorder can be food. If you relish a heavy and fatty meal at night just before sleeping, it is likely that it will keep you up during the night and you will be making trips to the kitchen to drink water. The opposite is also true that if you did not have anything to eat before sleeping then a hungry stomach can also keep you awake at night. So, make sure to have a light and healthy snack before going to bed. Other helpful and researched techniques to get a better good night sleep are to darken the room more and turn the face of clock away from you. If you are worried about something, get the stress out of your mind and onto a piece of paper. It will not only provide your mind with a clearer perceptive but it will also help you feel peaceful because you can now quit worrying about it. If you have a habit of stressing too much about even little things, then meditation is necessary for you.

Exercise can also get the job done for you. Exercise tires out your body a little bit and when you lay down after it, you instantly feel peaceful and immediately go to sleep because of the tiredness factor.

So, here is one other benefit of daily exercise on top of hundred others. Even after trying everything, you are unable to sleep soundly only then you should visit your doctor. Precaution is always better than medicine.

8) Avoid processed foods and sugars. Processed foods are unhealthy because they have already been deliberately changed before we consume them. Whenever the natural form of a food is altered, it is categorized as 'processed'. You have always been hearing it that eat fresh, eat healthy. Minimally processed foods can retain their physical and nutritional properties. These include bagged salads, frozen vegetables and meat. Then there comes some ready to eat foods. You must know that they have been through ultra-processing, as they have been formulated from oils, fats, sugar, salt, added flavors and preservatives. Always focus on eating fresh. No matter what you eat, if it is fresh, it is much less likely to cause any harm to your stomach. Many beverages recently present in the market have a label of protein drinks, energy drinks, sports drinks, sugar-free drinks. All of these are a scam.

They have high amounts of added sugars and hundreds of different chemicals and substituents. Any drink that says 'sugar-free' means something else is added beside the sugar. Otherwise the taste would be extremely bad and unbearable. They can add artificial flavors or some other types of processed sugar and it can hurt your digestive system badly. Because instantly they will create a sugar high for you and when your sugar level drops back, you again crave it.

Continuous consumption of sugar can never do your body any good. Prefer fresh juices, fruit juices and non-sugary beverages. Stay hydrated and let your body work at optimum levels.

9) Put away the salt shaker. A salt shaker at the dining table makes it too easy for you to consume excess salt. Excess salt can give you high blood pressure. So just pick the salt shaker up from the dining table and place it in a kitchen cupboard and only use it while preparing the meal. If you like spices or strong flavors in your food, you can add lime juice, garlic paste or red pepper flakes. Stock your fridge with fresh and dried herbs and use them instead of salt when needed. Blood pressure is the root cause for many different diseases and illnesses. It is also incurable. People that have the problem of blood pressure have reported that it stays with you throughout your life. You have to daily eat a pill in order to keep your blood pressure at a normal level. So, isn't it better that you avoid this problem altogether? Start eating meals with low amounts of salt and trust me, you will get used to the new taste in no time. It is not only healthy but also prevents you from spreading of terminal and fatal diseases. Just satiate on the existing level of salt present in the dish or meal you are going to eat.

10) Give yourself a break. Believe it or not, overtraining can turn out to be a problem. If your body is not given enough time to restore, it won't restore its health and ultimately your performance will decline day by day instead of getting better. There are symptoms that help you know that you are overdoing it and those symptoms are; moodiness, constant fatigue, lack of energy, depression and increased mental stress. A common complaint heard from people is that "no matter how much I do cardio exercises; I cannot seem to lose more than I have lost already". It is because you are working out too much. Just take a short step back, give your body time to relax and shorten your work out.

Another way to go around the problem is to divide and rule. If you do one hour of exercise, then divide it into two 30 minutes workout sessions; one in the morning and one in the evening.

This will prevent overtraining and will give your body time to rest in between. You can also start to work out on alternate days. For example, if you had a work out on Monday, then skip work out on Tuesday and have your next work out on Sunday. This will give time to your body that is enough for it to relax and restore its energy.

Always listen to what your body is telling you. Our bodies are well able to communicate with us, the problem is do we listen or not.

How does intermittent fasting prevent cancer?

Intermittent fasting helps to prevent cancer as well as it helps during its treatment. With each passing day, researches are being conducted on this matter and every day it proves further the fact that it does help in fighting cancer.

Prevention of cancer – Some research has shown that intermittent fasting fights cancer by lowering insulin resistance and levels of inflammation. Under the 'fasted state' of intermittent fasting, your body experiences lower insulin levels and tries to regain its energy by burning fats and excess calories. As a result of this process, toxins and damaged cells present inside the body also get automatically burned. Naturally, we would never know that there any damaged cells present inside our body that can induce our bodies to cancer. But intermittent fasting takes care of this problem on its own. It clears out all damaged and dysfunctional cells from our body which can later take shape of tumor or cancer.

This provides prevention from cancer.

How does intermittent fasting help to treat cancer? Intermittent fasting helps to boost the immune system which in return helps to fight the cancer that is already present. Treatment of cancer needs inner strength of the body so that it can fight it off. Intermittent fasting provides the body with enough power and stronger immune system and eventually it overcomes the cancer cells.

Another way cancer can help treating Intermittent Fasting is during chemotherapy. Fasting makes cancer cells more responsive towards chemotherapy and this helps to protect the remaining cells of the body. During chemotherapy, intermittent fasting greatly helps in *cellular regeneration.* It also protects all cells and our blood from the side-effects of chemotherapy. Chemotherapy has many other side-effects like fatigue, headaches and nausea. Intermittent fasting helps the body to deal with all these side-effects and in fact helps to prevent them from happening.

So, for existing cancer patients, intermittent fasting can help them to tolerate the pain and ailment during fighting cancer. It helps them in overcoming side-effects and also gives the rest of their body a protection from cancer. And for those who have a family history of cancer and are susceptible to have cancer in future are strongly recommended to intermittently fast. This will help them with prevention from cancer. They will continuously keep getting rid of dangerous and dysfunctional cells and this greatly improves the chances of preventing those cells to take on a form of cancer.

IF makes healthy eating simpler and easier

The best diet is the one with which you can stick to in the long-run. If intermittent fasting makes it easier and simpler for you to stick with a healthy diet plan then obviously you need to keep it as long as possible. It will help you with maintaining a healthy weight and also helps you to remain in a healthy condition. One of the main advantages of intermittent fasting is that it makes healthy eating simpler, easier and less time-consuming.

Other diet plans may require you to tediously work out your carb intake and limit the calorie intake for the day. This is not practical. You cannot assess your meal every time before you eat it. That's how intermittent fasting takes the edge over dieting plans. It does not require you to limit your food choices and calorie intake. It only helps you to maintain a healthy schedule of eating. Women who practice intermittent fasting, report that, intermittent fasting helped them to move from 3 meals to 2 meals a day. This made it easier for them to shift to a healthier lifestyle without drastically changing it. Intermittent fasting limits the "feeding window" of the day to few hours and this helps to move towards 2 meals a day plan. A gradual and steady shift in meals is important, so that your body doesn't go into a shock because of the new changes presented to it. Start from 3 meals and then gradually progress towards two meals. A diet is successful if it allows to you to remain consistent and doesn't demand sudden lifestyle changes. So, in short intermittent fasting is the best way to move to a healthier and easier lifestyle.

Chapter 6

Tips to ease through intermittent fast

Initially, you might find it hard to make it through the fast. It can be because you are not used to of staying hungry. Researches have put together a list of tips and strategies that will you ease through the fasting cycle.

Suppress your hunger with the help of green tea, black coffee and water. This is not a necessary step to implement during a fast; it's just for when you are experiencing an extreme hunger wave.

To satiate and suppress the hunger levels a little bit and ease through the fast; you can enjoy these drinks every once in a while.

Do not overdose on the amounts of these drinks and also don't drink them more than once or twice a day. Everything is bad when used in excess.

Try to listen and understand body cues. If you are feeling stress or anxiety without any significant reason, then it might be a cue from your body to relax. Feeling stressed in a fast is commonly observed especially during the initial days of fasting. this can often happen in certain periods of our lives.

This is not something to worry about but if it does not go away even after some time then it might be a signal from your body that it is getting exhausted.

Ease up on the hours of fasting and eat more nutritious dense foods.

Have healthy food available in the house. Foods with protein and veggies should be available in your home all the time. In this way, when you break your fast on a Sunday evening, you should be able to have a small healthy meal at home.

Eating out is not prohibited in intermittent fasting. But every once in a while, have a home-prepared healthy and fresh diet. When you have available options in home, you will automatically be tempted to cook something delicious and healthy. Also, when you have healthy foods available at home, you will be much less tempted to go out and eat unhealthy.

Clean out your fridge to avoid temptation. It might be already hard for you to make it through the fast and if you know that chocolates and pizza is present inside your fridge, then the temptation can cross the limits. So before starting a fast, clean out temptations from your fridge so that your focus is diverted from what to eat now.

Eat meals after a fast relatively slower. You might be tempted to go out and eat a heavy and big meal after your first fast in order to celebrate. But this will make you feel so exhausted and lazy for the rest of the day that you won't be able to get out of bed.

So, a useful tip is to go slow while eating meals after a fast because it will help you to eat just enough and you will feel energized for the rest of your day.

Meditate and indulge in light exercise. Initially, your focus during a fast will just be food. You will keep counting how many hours you have to go more without food and this can induce stress in your brain. So, in order to take your attention off from thinking about food, start meditation. It will divert your attention as well as bring peace to your body and rest of your day.

Light exercise helps to burn fat faster than anything. If your body allows you, then do indulge in light exercising. It will increase your physical fitness and will also increase the rate of weight-loss.

Eat plenty of whole foods on non-fasting days. Not everyone is looking to reduce weight through intermittent fasting.

Some people have a goal to get their body in a healthier condition than before. Even though fasting does involve staying away from foods for a certain portion of the day, it is still important to maintain a healthy eating style on the days when you are not fasting.

Eating healthy and whole foods will help you to stay away from all sorts of chronic illnesses as well as cancer. Whole foods include meat, eggs, fish, fruits and vegetables.

Stop, if you are feeling unwell. Having a sick feeling or generally feeling unwell is a sign that fasting is not your thing. It can also mean that your body is not ready for fasting right now.

If you feel unwell or sick, then stop, focus on healthy eating, increase nutrition and relax. Walk daily and slowly increase the time of walk so that your body can build higher stamina. Sometimes, you might have to help your body and this is one of those times.

Help your body to gain stamina and then when you feel healthy and energetic, you can try fasting again.

Re-evaluate your results. Try fasting for 7 days or 10 days before making a strong judgment call. You can try our 7-day guide that will help you make it through the initial 7 days of fasting.

After the specified time passes, if you still feel low on energy and a little light-headed then you need to ease up on fasting and choose another technique or formula of Intermittent Fasting. But if you feel great and active, then continue on your journey.

Research-proven advantages of IF for women

1) **Helps to regain hormonal balance.** Eating without any order and eating unhealthy can possibly induce an imbalance of hormones inside your body. If because of any reason, you are having a hormonal imbalance and are looking for easy ways to restore the balance, then intermittent fasting is the way to go. Research has proven that intermittent fasting helps restore the eating order. It specifies the times of

when to eat and when to stay hungry and it helps to maintain a healthy eating schedule. You may not realize the importance of eating at regular times but the women who are having the problem of hormonal imbalance; should be asked about its importance. Just follow intermittent fasting and it will restore balance of your hormones and will also take you to healthy eating schedules.

2) **Improves metabolism and insulin sensitivity.** Fasting induces low levels of insulin inside your body and when these levels are low; your body starts to gain energy from fats already present inside the body. So, higher insulin sensitivity means that your body easily goes to lower levels of insulin when fasting and thus starts to burn-off the fats. Another factor that contributes in the increase of insulin sensitivity is metabolic rate. If your metabolism is slow, you will be unable to digest the eaten meal quickly. It will take much longer for food to digest and thus won't give much time to your body to enter low insulin levels where it can burn-off fat. If you have a strong and fast metabolism, your body will process the food you ate much quicker and your body will remain under low insulin levels for higher time and thus burns higher amount of fat. In order to increase your insulin sensitivity, research has proven that it is beneficial to indulge in intermittent fasting, because it not only enhances your metabolism rate but also increases your body's sensitivity towards insulin levels.

3) **Improves eating patterns and hunger levels.** The research proven best advantage of intermittent fasting is its power to improve eating patterns. Intermittent fasting defines specific "eating periods" and "fasting periods". This helps to follow a timetable in eating. Eating at regular patterns has hundreds of proven benefits for the overall health of the body. It also helps with hunger levels. If you feel that

you never really feel hungry, that means that you don't give time to your body to digest and have another meal before the first one is digested. This causes adherence in entering fat-burning mode. You are eating regularly but you are not burning any fats. Fasting increases the hunger levels and helps your body to go into fat-killing mode. Therefore, if you are experiencing problems related to eating patterns or hunger levels, indulge in moderate intermittent fasting.

4) **Effective for weight-loss.** Many researches have been conducted on the important topic of "Does Intermittent Fasting really help to lose weight or not?" You will be pleased to know that intermittent fasting is worldwide recognized as a weight-loss method. It not only helps you lose weight but it also helps you to maintain your health while doing so. Diets mostly leave people with different kinds of nutritional and physical deficiencies but intermittent fasting has been proven to have no such side-effects. Intermittent fasting helps to increase insulin sensitivity which in return helps to lose weight because body starts to burn the fats inside the body. When the fats are burned, the next time you have a meal; it is used to fulfill the needs of the body and is not just stored as fat. Higher the fat-burn, lower the fat storage after the next meal and hence higher weight-loss.

5) **Improves brain function and makes immune system stronger.** Intermittent fasting has been proven to improve cognitive functions of brain and make brain activity fast. When you eat at regular patterns and at healthy, it provides healing powers to your entire body. The nutrition supplied helps to make all organs of the body to function better. Eating healthy and nutrition dense foods help you to build a stronger immune system. Immune system has to fight-off all bacteria and diseases. If it's not healthy then it cannot

provide your body the protection needed. Thus, to improve your immune system, you can opt for intermittent fasting.
6) **Fights diabetes and prevents cancer.** We already know that intermittent fasting helps with insulin sensitivity and keeps the insulin levels at a lower rate than normal. This proves that intermittent fasting can greatly help patients with diabetes. It keeps the sugar levels at moderate levels; not too high or too low. It also helps with prevention from cancer. Cancer is caused due to storage of dysfunctional and harmful cells. These cells need to be taken out of the body and intermittent fasting greatly helps with it. When you fast, your body is in a fat-burning and harmful cell removal process. That's how intermittent fasting helps to prevent cancer. Improves cellular regeneration and discards harmful cells.
7) **Intermittent fasting induces autophagy into your body.** Autophagy is a state in which body itself clears out junk from your body. Here junk is referred for harmful and useless cells inside your body that need to be taken out. It not only clears out such cells from your body but also helps in regeneration of new cells. Autophagy is a result of intermittent fasting. Without fasting, autophagy cannot be induced into the body naturally. Then you are left with chemotherapy only. So, in order to stay healthy and avoid medical procedures done on you, fast intermittently every now and then.
8) **Engages your mind and body.** Some people have complained about constant stress in their minds. And they claim that there are no obvious reasons for the stress. Mental stress can be caused by one of many reasons. It can be due to a workaholic nature, not resting enough, not eating enough, not eating healthy and never preparing healthy foods at home. Research has shown that when you

fast for a specific time and then enjoy a nutritious meal afterwards, it helps the brain to feel a sense of accomplishment. You will feel like you achieved something out of your day and this provides satisfaction to your mind. Meanwhile body is already engaged in taking care of excess fats, burning extra calories and sustaining its health and structure. Bu the end of the day, you will feel happy, enthusiastic and much more energetic. Engaging mind and body is necessary for a balanced body. So, intermittent fasting helps in another great way.

Reviews from women who practiced intermittent fasting

Surveys have been conducted and research has been undertaken to know about the reviews of women who practiced intermittent fasting. Reading these reviews can help you gain a clearer vision of what you can achieve by intermittent fasting, how did women successfully fasted and did they face any problems or not.

The overall reviews were positive and women highly appreciated and thanked for such a natural and easy to adopt technique.

The reviews are listed below in the form of general information so that it's easy for you to read it and judge for yourself if it's something you can achieve too or not.

Women who tried intermittent fasting for a week

After one week of practicing it, women reported that they definitely felt lighter. This doesn't mean they had a significant weight loss in a week.

It was just a way of expressing that they felt better and healthier than before. Some women said that weight-loss was little but negligible and some said they didn't have any weight-loss. Again, these results were after just one week and the body takes this much time just to adjust to fasting schedules.

They also reported about their appearance. One woman said that there was a loss of only quarter of an inch around her waist and there were no other significant changes seen. They also reported that by mid-week that is after 3 or 4 days of fasting, the dizziness and fogginess in their heads vanished due to fasting. And they didn't experience it any more after that.

These women said that the biggest advantage of intermittent fasting that we observed in a week was that it was an extremely easy and simple technique to follow. It adjusts well with anybody's lifestyle and doesn't require any drastic changes either.

It not only helped them regulate their eating patterns but it also made them eat healthy. They said that intermittent fasting schedules made them try and enjoy nutrient-dense foods and that's why within a week, they experienced feeling lighter and healthier than before.

This proves that intermittent fasting promotes and makes it easy to regulate eating patterns as well as puts you in a habit of eating healthy. This increases your health and fitness by a huge scale in a very short period of time.

Woman who tried intermittent fasting for 8 months

A woman who tried intermittent fasting was asked about her experience and her results and she openly communicated them so that all the women out there can know about the long-term effects of intermittent fasting. Her experience is described below.

She said that after college she injured and fractured her foot which caused her to stop exercising and even moving at all.

That's why she started with intermittent fasting because she wanted to maintain a healthy and fit body even though she could not exercise. After 7.5 to 8 months, she dropped almost 50 pounds, around 10% body fat and almost 40 inches all around her body.

And these were the results merely from intermittently fasting as she could do no walking or exercise. She was thankful for intermittent fasting because it helped her to get her BMI under the "normal' category. She said everybody asked her how she lost so much even when she could not exercise or walk.

She told everyone about her success due to intermittent fasting and also tried to bring them on this healthy technique too. She further said that the key to her success is **Consistency**.

She adopted the 4 days eat and 3 day fast schedule of intermittent fasting and never went any week without following this schedule.

The 3 days of fasting were non-consecutive and she made it clear many times. Women should not fast more than 24 hours and she followed the advice and it gained her the best possible results.

She had a little bit of difficulty in the starting week but this is something everyone faces. She saw that fasting had become easy for her before the first week even ended.

So, this gives many tips and tricks for all the women out there. If you want best results in a shorter time frame then there are a few things you need to consider.

First, find an intermittent fasting schedule suitable for you and stick to it. Second, you will have problems the first week like light-headedness or dizziness but don't worry; they will go away before or after one week.

Third, be consistent. Don't fast for one week and then stop fasting for the next week and then suddenly start fasting week after that.

This will induce an imbalance in your health, might even disturb your hormones and you will not be intrigued and willing to fast because your body is not being able to come under a habit of it.

Whatever schedule you pick, stick with it and stay consistent until the day you reach your goal-weight.

Conclusion

Final words on Intermittent Fasting for women

Fasting is natural – humans have been doing it since forever. The benefits of intermittent fasting greatly outweigh potential risks to it. These potential risks and dangers can only occur if you adopt fasting lifestyle without having ample knowledge about how fasting works and what are important considerations to keep in mind. To be further safe, you can also ask your doctor if it is healthy for you to fast or not. If you are not suffering from a chronic disease or specific medical conditions, then your doctor is most likely to give you the "go-ahead".

Intermittent fasting is a technique with various formulas. And you can try and adapt any of these formulas according to your lifestyle and preferences. You can take benefit from its many advantages like **weight-loss, disease prevention, better mental and physical performance and overall fitness and health.** Intermittent fasting allows you to choose your own fasting and feeding windows so that your body can optimally work and also meet its calorie needs. One picture of intermittent fasting that you don't want to be in is – you fast for 24 hours and then satisfy your hunger with binge-eating.

You also don't want to exceed the 24 hour specifies limit for women. Fasting is worth it because it will give you mental clarity in the morning before going to work. It does not affect your lifestyle. You can exercise according to your own desired intensity. You will sleep better and faster. And most important above all; you will lose a healthy amount of weight without it paralyzing your health!

Before getting started, try different schedules of fasting. Eat normally and then fast 1 or 2 times a week. Or fast and feast regularly in a day. Or fast every other day occasionally. Try out all these options before settling down with one formula of intermittent fasting.

Ease into intermittent fasting by starting from short fasting and eating windows. It will help you with initial hunger and discomfort. But if it becomes too uncomfortable, be honest with yourself and just take a step-back!

At the end of the day, nothing can have greater impact on your health than a lifestyle that prioritizes your mental, physical and emotional well-being. And a nutrition style that comprises of real whole foods not just empty carbs. No diet can offer you all of this in one package. But intermittent fasting is a gift for you with everything complimentary.

Intermittent Fasting for Women

© Copyright 2019 Jenna Dawson All rights reserved.

Written by Jenna Dawson

First Edition

Made in the USA
Columbia, SC
07 September 2019